Focus on Vision

FOCUS ON VISION

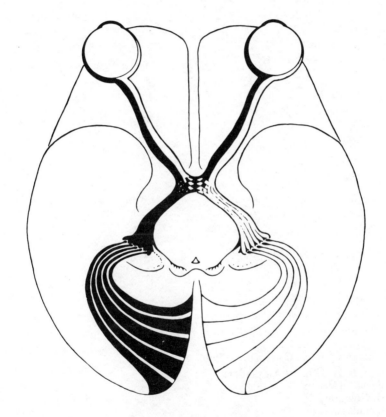

R. A. Weale

HARVARD UNIVERSITY PRESS

CAMBRIDGE, MASSACHUSETTS 1982

Library of Congress Cataloging in Publication Data
Weale, R. A. (Robert Alexander)
   Focus on Vision
   Bibliography: P
   Includes index
   1. Vision. I. Title.
   QP475.W34 1982   599'.01823   82-11974
ISBN 0-674-30701-1

First published 1982

Printed in Great Britain

Preface

In a sense, this book was written on request. David Hall told me that a paperback I had written a dozen or so years ago was popular with his students and ought to be brought up to date. Also it was out of print. I am afraid I look on bringing books up to date as an example of Achilles and the tortoise: time moves faster than the pen. Or even than the typewriter. On the other hand, just as I would not dream of giving the same lecture twice for fear that my boredom might infect that part of the audience that happens to be awake, I would be loathe to cover the same ground more than once in print. Not only the eye is bored by repetition. David Hall understood all that, and agreed that I might ring the changes, and concentrate on parts of the visual field that seemed particularly significant at the present time.

Admittedly, this involves an arbitrary choice, and neither inclusions nor omissions are always easy to justify. I owe it to the reader to give him a description of what the eye looks like, and how it is believed to work. He will be relieved, not insulted, to hear that there has been a lot of simplification without, I hope, the penalty of incoherence. That said, I thought that circadian aspects of visual activity might be of interest from a general biological point of view, and that the reader could take part in the tying up of a number of ends, inevitably left loose by the relative novelty of the topic. Age and development are hot issues also from a non-specialist point of view: it is, of course, easy to identify oneself with one topic or the other. Again, the stuff of ideas is made up of perceptions in one way or another. While I have to confess to scepticism as regards the prospects of the understanding of perception leading to one of thought, I do not believe the time has come to give up in the sense in which we no longer try to count the number of angels that can be accommodated on the tip of a pin. But the reader need not feel deprived: even though not exhaustive, the reading list is up to date. If the quartet before him makes him ask for more, the list will lead him to the sources without my intervention as a filter. Perhaps he will also understand what Achilles must have felt like.

RAW

I should like to thank Miss G. M. Villermet, for her endless help with illustrations, references, and keeping me in order; Miss R. Condliffe, for producing a typescript with fewer than the permissible number of grumbles; Mrs. S. Lawrence, for her ready assistance in the library; all at the Institute of Ophthalmology, University of London.

RAW

Contents

To Harris Ripps

1 The Window of the Soul

This is how Descartes defined the eye, unmindful that windows are looked out of, but looked into only by the rude. But the French philosopher had not failed to appreciate that the visual path is part of the two-pin system wherewith we are plugged into the world around us: the sensory or afferent side and the motor or efferent moiety which it controls.

This grossly simplified description summarizes the sequences of

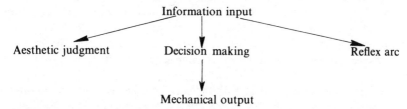

The research effort that has gone into studies of outer parts of these loops is understandably greater than is true of the central ones. The effects of 'noise' tend to accumulate, and so to obscure, the picture one obtains of the working, not to say, behaviour, of central stations of the system. In this context, 'noise' means a quasi response in any stimulated system capable of a response, there being no evident relation between the stimulus and the response. For example the crackling noise in an inferior record player is not due to modulations in the track (i.e. the stimulus) but to other unrelated, even if perhaps inevitable, causes.

Because we can not only study the visual system but are also able to see, vision has been probed in two ways one of which depends on the fact that it mediates perceptions while the other is independent of them. The two paths are often referred to as objective and subjective respectively. A horrible synonym for the latter, namely psychophysical, is used by an irresistible, if mistaken, majority. They are mistaken in the sense that physics linked to the soul (*psyche*), does not make sense. The basic difference is that, in objective experiments, the response of the visual path under test can, in principle, be recorded, whereas this is not the case when introspection is involved. For example, we can observe directly the retinal image formed of an outside object, and photograph it, just as we can display electric responses of the optic nerve on a television screen, and put them on video-tape. But we cannot record our impressions of size, brightness or colour without willing it. Of course, we must will to do any experiment that we decide shall be done. But a well-designed objective experiment assumes the inevitability of a reflex in a sense in which this is never true of one in which the answer depends on our introspection and a willingness to answer personal questions like 'Can you see this?'

Introspective studies can be subdivided, somewhat arbitrarily, into quantitative and qualitative ones. The former involve threshold judgments: e.g. they are
used to determine what marginal amount of radiation has to be added to one of
two equally irradiated surfaces to make one of them appear just noticeably
brighter. Note that this does not constitute a measurement of brightness (which is
impossible), but of an energy quantity or flux (cf. p. 6), which produces a
threshold difference in brightness. This brightness difference is not measured but
used as a criterion, just as the accuracy of alignment between a pointer and a line
on a scale is used as a criterion of a voltage or current measurement and not as a
measure of the magnitude of the electric units.

On the other hand, while a statement to the effect that the petals of a dandelion
are yellower than those of a pansy may be verifiable by other people, it is hard to
quantify. However, it is possible to agree on a scale of yellowness which need not
be uniform: it can be logarithmic or whatever, as long as its first differential e.g.
with respect to the concentration of a standard pigment remains positive or
negative. It is then possible to try and make a match between the perception of
one of the petal types and the perception of the variable yellow scale. If this
procedure is repeated with the other type of petal, it becomes possible to quantify
the difference between them in terms of some aspects of the visual stimulus they
produce.

It need hardly be stressed that, with the vast facilities that computers offer for
producing analogues of infinite arrays of stimulus points (but see p. 35), the above
principle of matching can be extended to a great variety of problems which,
though superficially qualitative, become amenable to quantification (Ch. 4).

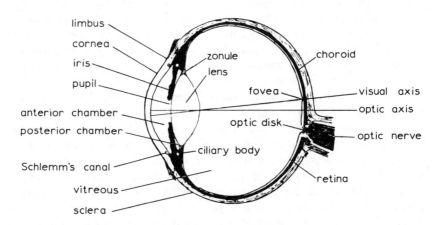

Fig. 1.1   A sagittal section through the human eye. (From Weale, 1968a. © 1968 Oliver
and Boyd, Edinburgh and London.)

The structure of the eye

The retina constitutes a great divide in this overall system. This light-sensitive
tissue that lines some 85 per cent of the inside of the eye-ball (Fig. 1.1) is, as it were,
the last stage at which functionally useful electro-magnetic energy from the

outside world can be detected. Here it is either absorbed or not. If not, it is wasted, potentially heating, if not actually damaging, nearby tissues. But if absorbed in the retinal photo-receptors it is potentially active and may elicit a visual message. It is plain that, even before reaching the retina, the incident radiation traverses several tissues with which it may interact. These are the glassy cornea, the liquid aqueous, the highly vascular iris, the crystalline lens, which is merely an aid to focusing, and the jelly-like vitreous humour more than 99 per cent of which consists of water.

The interaction between radiation and these tissues is strictly optical and fulfils no function from the point of view of initiating any nervous message. Typical negative feed-back mechanisms exist in this system: once initiated, the nervous message may influence the iris and thereby vary the pupillary diameter. It may also serve to control tension in the suspensory ligaments which hold the lens in position. We shall see later that this may serve to modify the shape of the lens and therewith its optical focus or power. While the outer cornea is the principal image-forming device, the lens provides, as we just noted, a fine focusing device, enabling well-defined retinal images to be formed of distant and near objects in turn. It is obvious that, without this capacity, an eye normally geared for distance as is true of that of man, could not have allowed evolutionary pressure to develop the manual dexterity which has given him control of his world.

The properties, like the diseases, of the dioptric apparatus are of importance insofar as they affect image formation, image contrast, and image intensity. The first is determined by the curvature of the component surfaces of the optic media and, of course, by the relevant refractive indices. The second remains optimal only if the media, notably the crystalline lens, are clear: this is to say, they have to be free of scattering loci or opacities. Such utter freedom is rare. If a pinhole is made in an opaque card, light admitted through it into each eye in turn, and the aperture moved about, then one can sometimes detect a refractive inhomogeneity manifested by an irregular movement of the narrow pencil of light that scans the

Fig. 1.2 Light micrograph of the human cornea from 27-year-old male. Bar = 100 nm. (From Marshall and Grindle, 1978. © 1978 *Trans. Ophthal Soc. U.K.*)

pupil of the eye. Lastly, image intensity is determined by the optical absorbance of the ocular media. Let us turn to each of these factors in a little more detail.

The cornea

The cornea consists of four layers, namely an outer epithelium, Bowman's membrane, the stroma, and Descemet's endothelium (Fig. 1.2). The stroma is made up of individual fibres and were it not for their pseudo crystalline arrangement, it would be opaque. The diameter of the adult cornea is about 11 mm. What is optically of more significance is its radius of curvature R: at the optical centre, in practice the central 3 mm, it is 8 mm (Emsley, 1955), but increases towards the corneal border or limbus to about twice this value. Optical power being expressed in dioptres (D; one dioptre is the power of a lens with a focal length f equal to 1000 mm: hence number of dioptres = 1000/f), and the refractive index μ of the corneal stroma being approximately equal to that of water (1.33) the power of the normal cornea is $1000/f = 1000\,(\mu - 1)/R = +40D$. As the refractive power of the human eye is roughly $+60D$, we have here the justification for the above statement regarding the importance of the cornea as an image-forming device. The balance ($\sim +20D$) is taken up by the lens. However, its power is variable, and can be increased by a mechanism first elucidated by Helmholtz (1855) (p. 17).

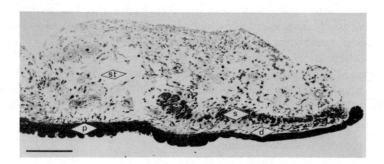

Fig. 1.3   Radial section through iris: st, stroma; s, sphincter; d, dilator; p, pigment epithelium, Bar = 100 nm. (Original: courtesy J. Marshall, Institute of Ophthalmology.)

The iris

The next optically significant part is the pupil. This is a variable aperture in the iris, its area being controlled by the mutually antagonistic actions of two reflexly innervated muscles (Fig. 1.3). One of these consists of fibres that surround the aperture: on contraction, they reduce its area. The sphincter, as it is called, is counteracted by the dilator, the fibres of which are radial. When they contract, e.g. in the dark or during apprehensiveness or emotional arousal, the pupil dilates. We see, therefore, that it determines the quantity of light reaching the retina, and is clearly one of the factors to be controlled when retinal irradiation has to be measured e.g. in threshold determinations (cf. p. 81).

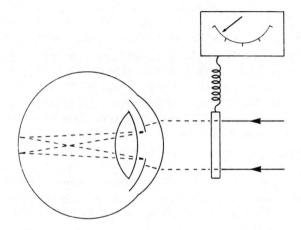

Fig. 1.4   To show that the measurement of the irradiance of the retina for the intact eye is done by determining the intensity incident on the cornea. Allowance has to be made for the effect of the pre-receptoral media if the *retinal* irradiance is to be estimated.

The crystalline lens

In addition to its ability to vary the overall power of the eye, the crystalline lens also modifies retinal irradiance. The reason is that, in a number of species it is coloured: in man, it is yellow. This is due to its absorption of short wavelength radiation. The absorbance has to be known or estimated if a value for the retinal irradiance is to be derived from radiometric measurements at the point of entry into the eye (Fig. 1.4). Its value can vary from person to person, and does so fairly systematically as a function of age (Ch. 3).

Retinal illumination

The above factors enable one to form an estimate of the retinal irradiance due to any object the intrinsic 'brightness' I of which is known. Let us assume that such an object is so far away from the eye (distance = D) that the illumination due to it in the pupillary plane is uniform. Let its area be A'. Then if an intensity I is radiated into space per unit area of the radiator (unit: candela), and if the inverse square law holds and one candela emits light into one solid angle (unit: lumen) then the irradiance in the pupil plane will be $IA'/4\pi D^2$ (unit: lumen/sq cm). The pupil area α (projected into a plane perpendicular to the incident radiation) intercepts $IA'\alpha/4\pi D^2$. Given that the posterior nodal distance of the eye (cf. Emsley, 1955) is equal to d, the size of the retinal image of the radiator is equal to $A'' = A'd^2/D^2$. If no absorption occurs, the amount of radiation reaching the retina per unit time per unit area is consequently $I\alpha/4\pi d^2$ (unit: troland). Note that the only variables are the emittance of the object and the pupil area. In practice losses occur in the dioptric apparatus owing to spectral absorption. Let the transmissivities of the cornea, aqueous, lens and vitreous be given by T(C), T(Q), T(L), and T(V) respectively; then the retinal irradiance I(Ret) becomes attenuated as their maximum values are less than 100 per cent. However, I(Ret) is further reduced in the central parts of the retina by a factor T(M), where M stands for macular pigment. This is a yellow carotenoid substance which, together with the yellow coloration of the crystalline lens may serve to minimize chromatic aberration in the human eye. A fraction of the light entering the eye is also reflected from its back, the fundus oculi, which has a reflectivity R. It follows that the maximum amount *available* to the retina is equal to

$$I(Ret) = I\alpha\{[T(C)\ T(Q)\ T(L)\ T(V)\ T(M)\ (1+R)]/4\pi d^2\}$$

due allowance being made for the spectral variations of all the quantities except α (but see below). The significance of this expression is that, given a knowledge of the expression in { } (Fig. 1.5), the retinal irradiance can be calculated from extra-ocular measurements.

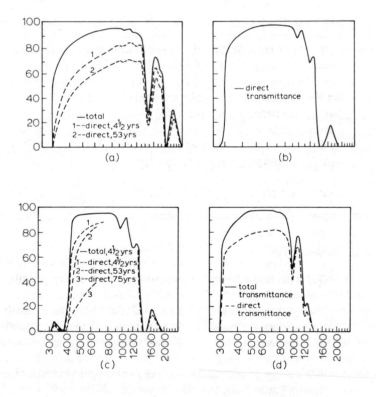

Fig. 1.5a *Ordinate*: spectral transmissivity (%) of the dioptric media of the human eye; *abscissa*: wavelength in millimicrons (1 mμ = 1 nm). a: cornea; b: aqueous humour; c: crystalline lens; d: vitreous humour. 'Total' means transmittance measured over a wide angle, 'direct' over a narrow one. (After Boettner and Wolter, 1962.)

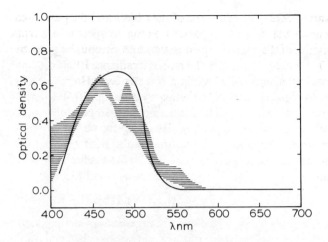

Fig. 1.5b The shaded area shows the range of various estimates for the optical density (absorbance) of the human macular (yellow) pigment. The curve represents the absorbance of a hypothetical filter, so computed as to minimize chromatic aberration and to maximize overall spectral transmission. (After Reading and Weale, 1974.)

In practice, the above treatment involves a simplification valid in many cases. It ignores aberrations and diffraction. These are dealt with in texts on physical optics, and here occupy points of interest insofar as they show how the eye combats them. The severest defect is spherical aberration. This is the designation of the fact that parallel pencils of light entering an aperture near its periphery are brought to a focus nearer to the image-forming surface than is true of the central points. Image definition is affected adversely as the pencils from a given point on the object do not meet in a single point, as rigid geometry would demand, but in a cusp.

The eye counteracts the adverse effects of spherical aberration in four ways:

(a) The periphery of the cornea is flatter than is its centre: this diminishes the refraction of the peripheral pencils.

(b) When the eye accommodates the crystalline lens for near vision (cf. pp. 17 and 132), and the visual axes converge so that diplopia (or double vision) may be avoided, the pupil constricts reflexly. Consequently only the central pencil of light is admitted to the retina.

(c) The refractive index of the crystalline lens is maximal at its centre, namely the nucleus: hence, even when the pupil is unconstricted – as is true in the dark – the refraction of the peripheral pencils is attenuated in relation to that of the central ones.

(d) Finally as shown by Laties (1969), the axes of the primate retinal photo-receptors are not directed radially but point approximately toward the pupil (Fig. 1.6). This has two effects. By virtue of their directional properties (p. 20) this enables them individually to respond preferentially to rays passing directly through the pupil to the detriment of stimulation e.g. by light scattered in the lens or the eye in general. Secondly, a beam coming to a focus on a surface other than

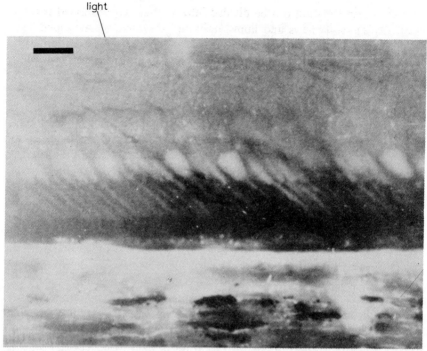

Fig. 1.6 Photo-receptor orientation in the superior vertical meridian of a squirrel monkey eye beyond the equator toward the ora serrata; the inclination away from the perpendicular is over 40°. Freeze-dried, unfixed, directly embedded eye. Bar = 2μ. Interference contrast microscopy. (From Laties, 1969. © Longman Group Ltd, Harlow.)

the retina shares attributes with scattered light. If, therefore, an object emits a beam focused by the centre of the optics, and also other beams defocused by spherical aberration, then the focused moiety will provide the more effective of the two stimuli.

It will be noticed that, from an operational point of view, factors (a) and (c) have characteristics of repair processes whereas (b) and (d) have the attributes of surgery: what is harmful is removed. Chromatic aberration, which is due to refraction being a spectral variable, is counteracted only by optical surgery. The eye is focused optimally for (green) radiations in the neighbourhood of 550 nm The consequent defocusing of longer wavelengths is not serious, but that of short ones is. In point of fact the aberration across the spectrum amounts to 1.5 D, and the major part of this occurs at short wavelengths. Classical optics knows of only two ways of producing achromatic imaging: by means of either spherical mirrors or lens doublets (or triplets) with components having different refractive indices. These methods are not surgical but conservative, and not used in the eye. The latter uses the spectral filters mentioned on p. 9.

A sideways step

It is useful to think of filters not just e.g. in terms of sunglasses, but in a more general way which is helpful in sorting out various aspects of the visual process. In the most general terms, a filter is a device used for modifying the transmission of information. Information can be divided into wanted and unwanted parts. If someone tells us some news, and 'hums' and 'hahs', these inarticulate sounds tend to get ignored as we concentrate on his message. When the unwanted information is random, the communication engineer refers to it as noise. But this is merely a special case of unwanted information (cf. p. 35). A filter serves to increase the proportion of the wanted information in the total information flux. This implies that its characteristics are always expressible as a pure fraction, and that it is useless if the fiducial figure is 100 per cent. In general, a comparison is made between the ratio of the information flow passed by the filter and that incident on it. It follows that a filter acts on a spectrum in the broadest sense of the word. A horizontal bar may act as a filter for cars less than 150 cm in height. A sieve is a filter for transverse areas. A loudspeaker is a filter for audio-frequencies. A ticket machine is a filter for money.

Returning to chromatic aberration, we noted that it is radiation of short wavelengths that is specifically defocused, and therefore unwanted. If it can get preferentially absorbed before stimulating the retina, the ratio of wanted to unwanted radiation will be increased. Two filters are available to fulfil this objective. We have met them on p. 6 as attenuators in general, namely the yellow crystalline lens and the yellow macular pigment. In white (day-) light, they appear yellow because the complementary blue and violet parts of the spectrum are preferentially absorbed. They act remarkably well as compensators for chromatic aberration. However, there is another remedy for chromatic aberration, and this lies within the percipient elements of the retina. If one measures the threshold of the fovea with spectral lights it is found that it is relatively low – i.e. the sensitivity high – in those parts of the spectrum where chromatic aberration is minimal. But sensitivity is low (Fig. 1.7) where chromatic aberration is high. This drives home another point worth making in connection with filter theory: there is no need to filter out information that the sensor cannot

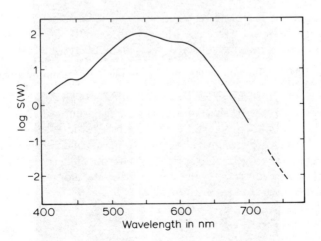

Fig. 1.7 Weighted spectral sensitivity function for the fovea. All the test-fields were 45′ in size or smaller. (From Ripps and Weale, 1976. © Academic Press Inc., New York and London.)

detect. In other words, filters and sensors act multiplicatively. In the case of the fovea lacking sensitivity to short wavelengths, it reinforces the actions of the pre-receptoral filters.

Diffraction cannot be classed with optical aberrations because it is due to the nature of light. There is no way of correcting a system for this defect of the image in the same sense in which one cannot correct gravity. The theory of diffraction is abstruse, and one of the significant points applicable to the eye is the following. The image of a point object such as a star cannot be dimensionless. Granted that some parts of the diffraction pattern are brighter than others, and an inadequately responding sensor may reproduce only the most intense part of the pattern (Fig. 1.8a): it can be shown however, that the resulting pseudo-point image is incomplete, and consequently fails to convey parts of the information that are latent. The complete pattern is described in a telling manner by the so-called point-spread function.

It can be shown, on the basis of a number of verified assumptions, that if a plane monochromatic electro-magnetic wave passes through a narrow slit, each part of the slit can be pictured to act as a point source of radiation. Since radiation is transmitted by transverse waves the amplitudes of all the spherical ripples will combine: if two points in diffraction space are both positive or negative they will add; if equal and opposite they will cancel each other. The overall addition of the amplitudes of all the elements results in the pattern shown in Fig. 1.8b. The

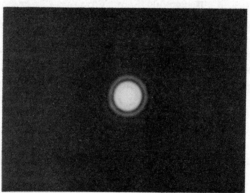

Fig. 1.8a   Diffraction pattern produced in light of 550 nm by a pinhole.

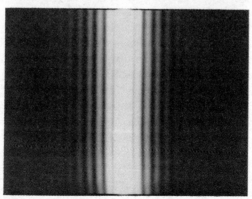

Fig. 1.8b   Diffraction pattern produced in light of 550 nm by a narrow slit.

separation of the diffraction bands is inversely proportional to the width of the slit, and to the wavelength of the radiation but approximately proportional to the distance between slit plane and display plane of the diffraction pattern. When the slit is rotated in its plane about its centre, we obtain a circular aperture, and it is possible to imagine Fig. 1.8a as derived from Fig. 1.8b. We conclude therefore that, given that 'white light' consists of the sum of monochromatic radiations as Newton demonstrated in Trinity College, Cambridge, almost three centuries ago, all images consist of the superposition of diffraction patterns. However, these can be detected only when the ratio of aperture diameter D to the distance of the display plane is small, in practice of the order 0.05 rad or less. In the eye, f is 17 mm hence an artificial pupil less than 2 mm in diameter facilitates the perception of diffraction bands (cf. p. 13 for the resolving power of the eye). An artificial pupil may be needed because the normal young pupil does not usually constrict to a diameter smaller than some 3 mm.

We have earlier referred to the spread function of an image. It describes intuitively what is observed – namely the failure of an optical system to concentrate energy within the dimensionless confines of a geometrical point. There is, however, another way of describing an image, which is mathematically convertible to the above. It is based on the notion of spatial frequency. In order to savour fully the elegance of this approach, familiarity with Fourier analysis (Hsu, 1970) is indispensible. But the underlying principles are easily stated.

It is best to view any image, indeed even any object, as an amplitude mountain range. This is to say, we imagine planes perpendicular to the image plane and plot along them vertical measures proportional to the amplitude of the luminous intensity (Fig. 1.9). Thus, if we make a comparison with maps, we see the image in terms of contour lines, but wish to think of it as a plaster relief, with amplitudes replacing the plaster. The bottom part of Fig. 1.9 represents a section along the plane AB in the upper part, and shows the amplitude mountains and valleys. Now the Fourier approach to this mountainscape is based on the idea that the outline can be described mathematically in terms of spatial waves one of which is indicated with the broken curve. It is evident that such a simple (sine or cosine) wave mimics the outline only crudely. However, it can be shown that the addition of other waves with different wavelengths λ/n, where n is an integer, and varying amplitudes can provide a useful approximation to this or any other outline. The accuracy with which this can be done depends on the number of individual wave-trains that are employed: perfect matching being obtained only with an infinity of trains. Sharp amplitude contours require the presence of short-wavelength trains. Frequency is the reciprocal of wavelength and has some advantages over that term: we say, therefore, that sharp amplitude contours have a large high-frequency component. It follows that Fig. 1.9, as is true of any image, can be transsected in any direction. More sensibly, it can be analysed, line by line, in a horizontal or a vertical sense and the Fourier frequency sums can be determined for each of them. The original image can be reconstructed from this information.

If we return for a moment to Fig. 1.8 we can see that this is represented relatively simply by a number of spatial wave-trains. We note also that the more widely the bands are spaced, the lower the frequencies that are needed. But we also noted that a small pupil (or narrow slit) leads to a widely spaced pattern. The conclusion is that, since a point object can be represented only by an infinite sum of frequencies ranging from 0 to ∞, the slit or pupil transmits only low spatial frequencies.

Higher frequencies are cut off, and the so-called cut-off frequency q_c at which this occurs for coherent radiation is given approximately by the expression

$$q_c = r/\lambda d$$

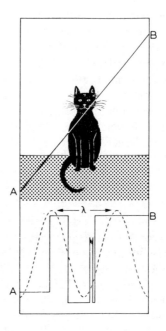

Fig. 1.9 A measurement of the light intensity along $\overline{AB}$ reflected from the above picture might yield approximately the continuous curve shown in the lower part of the figure. The dashed sine-curve analytically describes the continuous curve to a very rough extent. Its spatial frequency f may be defined as $1/\lambda$, where λ is half the width of the frame. The addition of different amounts of curves having frequencies 2f, 3f, etc. refines this approximation. This process can be repeated for other lines till a group of equations is obtained which describes the picture with such fidelity that a reasonable reproduction can be made from it. This type of analysis is also useful for the study of the imaging and reproducing power of the human visual system.

where r is the radius of an image-forming aperture d units away from a diffracting discontinuity emitting radiation of wavelength λ. Now it can be shown that the RHS of the above expression is equal to $n_0 \sin \theta_0 / 0.5 \lambda_0$ for incoherent radiation, the suffix relating to object space, $\sin \theta_0$ being the semi-angular aperture of a lens system of focus f or $\sin \theta_0 \approx (r/f) (1 - r^2/2f^2)$. This can be applied to the eye. However, as the retina is usually not directly accessible for measurement, retinal distances are more conveniently expressed in terms of visual angles: these are equal to retinal angles when referred to the ocular nodal points. Since the posterior nodal distance ~ 17 mm, 1 mm on the retina is equivalent to $3.37°$. Thus if $\lambda_0 = 5.5 \times 10^{-4}$ mm, and we assume a pupil diameter of 3 mm, then only periods greater than about 0.5 minutes of arc will be transmitted by the ocular dioptrics. In fact, the observed value is more nearly 1' although the upper limit is not infrequently reached. Note that, the above expression is formally similar to that for the diameter D of the first Airy disk, namely

$$D = 1.22\ F\lambda$$

from which it differs in the magnitude of the constant term. F is the numerical aperture, equal to $f/2r$. It is to be emphasized that the relation for the cut-off frequency holds only when the performance of the eye is limited by the diffraction of light. If, for some reason, the pupil is increased, the performance of the lens (see below) is no longer 'diffraction limited', but governed by the spherical and other aberrations of the dioptric system.

The latter play a relatively minor role when an image is formed with monochromatic (coherent) radiations from a laser. If such light is used in an interferometer, fringes are obtained which can be used in testing visual resolution in a manner analogous to that described below.

Contrast

The visual world does not, however, consist of just black and white in spite of Fig. 1.9. It contains many grey areas. In general, contrast varies from place to place. Even in a mathematically simple arrangement, such as a grating, it is essential to consider not just the periodicity but also its modulation. To return to our mountainous analogy, this is a measure of the amplitudes (or altitudes) of peaks and valleys respectively. If the luminous intensity at point A in Fig. 1.10 is I_G and at point B, I_B, then the intensity contrast can be given by

$$C = (I_G - I_B)/(I_G + I_B) = -(1 - I_G/I_B)/(1 + I_G/I_B).$$

It is, as ever, important to be clear whether one is dealing with intensity or amplitude contrast. C varies within limits of 0 and 1. It can, of course, be positive or negative, depending on the relative magnitudes of the contrasting quantities.

The immediately practical significance of contrast, insofar as the eye is concerned, relates to focusing. If we adjust a lens, a microscope, a camera for 'focus' – when this is not done automatically – we maximize the contrast of an image. Granted we look for a 'sharp' edge, i.e. high spatial frequencies: we shall see why below. But we try to turn dark greys into blacks and light greys into whites, and accept that setting as the in-focus one for which this difference is maximal and, incidentally, unique in the sense in which out-of-focusness is not. A line looks blurred on either side of the image plane of an image-forming device.

The quality of such a device is readily described in terms of the above concept as applied to various spatial frequencies: and this also applies to the eye. Suppose we image Fig. 1.10 by means of a lens system on a screen or, for brevity's sake, on the face of some scanning radiometer which can determine the luminous intensity at any point of the secondary image. It is then possible to determine its modulation or contrast. Let it be C". As we already know the value for the primary image C', we can define the modulation transfer of the lens system in terms of C''/C'. If this ratio M is unity, the system is perfect, or, preferably, lossless. In general, the value of M varies inversely with spatial frequency: i.e. lens systems are spatial frequency filters (cf. p. 9). A curve giving M as a function of the spatial frequency is called a modulation transfer function (MTF). A system free from aberrations is diffraction limited: consequently M drops to zero at the cut-off frequency q_c.

Several workers have obtained values for the MTF of the human eye by studying retinal images of external objects. This can be done either directly with the use of sinusoidal gratings or via the determination of the line-spread function, as indicated on p. 10. When the MTF is expressed logarithmically its zero-value is indeterminate, but a value between $\bar{2}$ and $\bar{3}$ is practically indistinguishable from the theoretical limit.

Fig. 1.10   The analysis illustrated in Fig. 1.9. is achieved more easily by means of a sinusoidal light distribution than by the use of cats. A typical study involves the determination of the just noticeable contrast (p. 15) for different frequencies (cf. Fig. 1.11).

The above instrumental method for studying the optical quality of the eye has been frequently and successfully replaced with a measurement of the spatial contrast threshold (or sensitivity) function. The procedure is simple. A grating of variable contrast and spatial frequency is generated electrically and displayed on a television screen. The absolute frequency depends, of course, on the viewing distance. The observer varies the contrast till it reaches threshold. The data obtained for various frequencies show a high sensitivity (low threshold) for low spatial frequencies and *vice versa* (Fig. 1.11). They vary systematically with luminance level. Note that the cut-off frequency q_c drops with luminance. Since q_c is proportional to pupil diameter (p. 12), and the pupil diameter varies inversely with the luminance owing to the operation of the light reflex, no optical

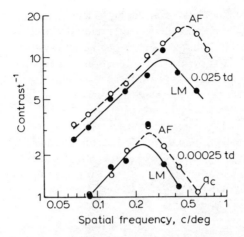

Fig. 1.11 *Ordinate*: reciprocal of contrast threshold as determined by two observers at retinal illuminations shown. *Abscissa*: Spatial frequency, c/°. The test-grating subtended at the eye an angle of 50° and was varied centrally, a faint red spot ensuring fixation. (After Fiorentini and Maffei, 1973.)

explanation can at present be advanced for this observation. However, we have to remember that the grating pattern covers a retinal area at least 1 or 2 mm square in area. Thus the linear angular subtense is of the order of 3°–6° of visual angle. At low luminance levels the central, foveal part of the retina, where visual resolution is optimal, reduces its response: vision is mediated essentially by non-foveal receptors, namely the rods. The spatial frequency spectrum of the rod-mechanism is much curtailed at the high-frequency end of the spatial spectrum. The explanation of the above conundrum is to be sought, therefore, not in the optics of the system but in its response mechanism.

A considerable literature has grown up on the basis of the above elements of image analysis, but it would take us too far to dwell on the many interesting off-shoots. We shall observe below that there are aspects of cerebral image analysis which are easiest to understand if approached from the point of view of Fourier analysis.

Accommodation

However, it also facilitates the understanding of an important reflex, namely how the eye (a) assesses when an image is in focus, and (b) how it focuses out-of-focus images. In classical parlance an image is in focus when it is 'sharp': in the light of the above considerations it is 'sharp' when it has a large content of high spatial frequencies. High means in this context 50–60 c/°, since this represents the upper limit of what the eye can resolve. It is easily seen that, if one were to move a screen from the image plane of a lens along the optic axis toward the lens, the amplitude of the higher frequencies would progressively diminish: in the lens plane the transfer function would be zero as the illumination on the screen would be uniform, no component of the spatial frequency spectrum of the object having a

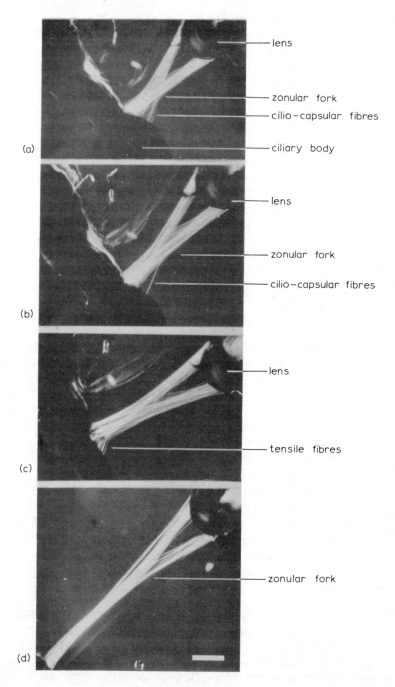

Fig. 1.12 Preparation of whole zonular system (sagittal section with region of ora serrata top left). The lens (♂ aet 37) appears tipped backwards by some 70° and exerts mild tension on the zonule, which therefore gradually peels away from the ciliary body (a–d). Note the zonular fork and the cilio-capsular amplifier fibres which are gradually torn off. (c) shows the appearance of tensile fibres. Bar = 1 mm. (After Rohen and Rentsch, 1969.)

measurable amplitude in this plane. Similarly, if the screen were moved from the image plane of the lens so as to increase its distance from the latter, the MTF would diminish and reach zero at infinity. We see therefore that the operational description of the image plane is that for which a given object–lens disposition gives a maximum value for the MTF.

Now, if the brain does not know the spatial frequency content of the object, it can assess the maximum possible value of that of the image only if it employs a scanning device, that is to say if, in principle, it hunts for the high frequencies in the manner described above. This is why Fry (1955) has stressed that the stimulus to the mechanism of accommodation (focusing of the lens) is the blur of an image. This is a subjective description of a spatial high-frequency deficit. Phillips and Stark (1977) have shown that blur is a sufficient stimulus in that accommodation is stimulated no matter whether it is the object (e.g. in the form of a projected image) or the retinal image that is out of focus.

The functional anatomy of the mechanism of accommodation was first elucidated by Helmholtz and refined during the last 125 years. In primates the crystalline lens is normally adjusted 'for distance': in a normal (emmetropic) eye, an object at infinity will then be focused on the retina. The precise position is still a matter for contention. The lens is held in this adjustment by the tension in the suspensory ligaments (Fig. 1.12) whereby it is attached to the inner anterior aspect of the eye. The fibres, collectively known as the zonule, terminate (Fig. 1.13) on the one hand near the equatorial region of the capsule – which contains the lenticular bulk – and, on the other, in the substance of the ciliary muscle. Like all involuntary muscles the latter consists of smooth unstriated fibres: they run in a posterio-anterior direction and then separate from the wall of the globe to follow a course along a circle perpendicular to the axis of the eye. This is why, for a long time, two muscles were thought to be involved in the accommodative process. The muscle contains elastic elements which expand when the muscle fibres contract.

When innervated via the neuro-muscular junctions, the muscle fibres contract. Consequently, the muscular mass moves anteriorly and centripetally so that the tension on the zonule is reduced. The elastic energy stored in the lens matrix is therefore released with the result that the lens bulges: its optical power is increased and objects nearer than infinity – in practice less than 6 m away – can be sharply focused on the retina. When accommodation is relaxed the above-mentioned elastic elements return the muscular bulk to its unaccommodated form; they pull on the zonule, flatten the capsule which acts by compression against the elastic lens matrix, and the lens returns to its minimum power.

Such a sequence of events is elicited only if foveal vision is involved. This is hardly surprising since it is the only part of the eye that responds to high spatial frequencies. Although the focused retinal image outside the fovea may also contain them, if the sensing mechanism does not respond to them they might just as well not exist (pp. 9, 45). Our understanding of the system was much advanced by Campbell's observation (1960) to the effect that the state of accommodation of the unstimulated eye is not stationary, but exhibits micro-fluctuations with an amplitude of approximately 0.1 D and a temporal frequency of 0.5 c/s. He demonstrated convincingly that these were not a manifestation of instrumental noise, since they occurred synchronously in both eyes. It follows that their origin

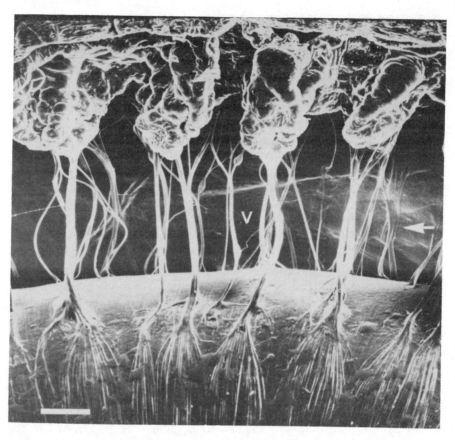

Fig. 1.13   The anterior equatorial region of the lens, the zonule, the anterior face of the vitreous (V), and the anterior end of the ciliary processes. The posterior zonular fibres lie upon, and seem to adhere to, the anterior surface of the vitreous (arrow). The anterior zonular fibres insert near the anterior end of the ciliary processes. Bar = 0.2 mm. (From Davanger, 1975. © Scriptor Publisher ApS. Copenhagen.)

is central. Qualitatively they may be interpreted as follows: in adults the power of the lens varies within the limit of ± 2 D searching for maximum contrast at high spatial frequencies. This scanning enables the accommodative loop to latch onto the conditions that maximize the MTF. When the pupil diameter is reduced to pinhole dimensions, the requisite high frequencies are not transmitted by the system and accommodation fails: with a pupil even 1 mm in diameter, $q_c \simeq 32\,\text{c}/°$ (cf. p. 12). We see that this approach offers a crude but informative view on accommodative control.

A refinement involves the careful dynamic control of the stimulus, and the servo-aspect of accommodation was studied by Stark *et al.* (1965). They stimulated the system periodically, and showed that the mechanism is helped by a 'prediction operator', which enables a hunting or scanning system to home onto its position of equilibrium – in this instance, in-focusness. By using a large dilated 7 mm pupil, and an artificial 1 mm one, it was possible to distinguish the closed-loop from the open-loop condition: a small pupil eliminates the need for accommodation. It turned out that the former attenuates a lot of noise falling within the effective bandwidth of the lens feed-back control system. The closed loop shows a peak when the stimulation alternates at 2 c/s. This must depend *inter alia* on the elastic properties of the system.

Photo-receptors

As mentioned earlier, the accommodation reflex is mediated by the fovea, the centre of which is populated exclusively by cones. At about 0.15 mm from the fixation area (FA) the first rods make their appearance, and then, contrary to that of the cones, their spatial density increases to a maximum at between 3 and 6 mm from FA (Østerberg, 1935). The spatial density of the cones decreases progressively toward the anterior limit of the retina, the ora serrata. There is no hypothesis to explain the peculiar doughnut shaped distribution of the rods. At 120 000 000 per retina they heavily outnumber the 6 000 000 cones and remind us that our eyes are basically instruments for nocturnal use. They have collectively a threshold lower than that of the cones by some four orders of magnitude (cf. Ch. 2), even though, receptor for receptor, the thresholds are of the same order (Fig. 1.14). The cones mediate colour vision and, as we noted above, have the higher cut-off frequency at normal levels of illumination.

The receptors share a peculiarity first pointed out by Laties (1969) as a result of a remarkable embedding technique he developed for the study of primate eyes (cf. p. 20). The latter were e.g. embedded in Epon after being pre-treated in different ways, which included freeze-drying without fixation (cf. p. 90). The hardening of the ocular tissues resulting from this treatment reduced the effects of

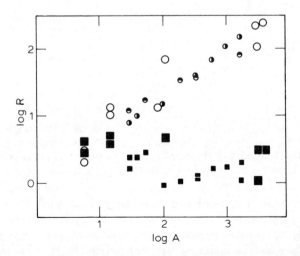

Fig. 1.14   Log ratio of foveal to extra-foveal thresholds in the dark-adapted human eye as a function of the test-area in log square minutes of arc. *Circles*: ratios expressed in terms of intensities. *Squares*: the corresponding values expressed in terms of 'effective stimuli' which take account of retinal summation. Different symbols relate to different authors. (After Weale, 1958.)

mechanical deformation and shear, which would otherwise invalidate conclusions one may draw from the relative positions of ocular layers and their
components. The receptors were clearly revealed by epi-illumination microscopy
and seen not to be pointing along ocular radii (Fig. 1.6, 1.15), but to include
angles with them that increased with the distance from the fovea. This was later
formalized (Laties and Enoch, 1971), and does not appear to be typical just of
primate retinae. The function of this pupillo-petal arrangement, which appears to
be the result of foetal development and not of any post-natal phototropism, is to
maximize the efficiency of the conversion of radiation into chemical action. We
shall see below (p. 24) that vertebrate receptors are 'triggered' by the minimum
amount of energy when the latter travels parallel to their axes. There is an
interesting phenomenon, known as the Stiles–Crawford effect, illustrating this.
If two thin equally intense pencils of light, directed at the fovea, enter the eye, one
through the pupillary centre, the other near its edge, then the central pencil
appears more effective than any other (Fig. 1.16). This effect seems more marked
for cones than for rods, but this is still open to argument.

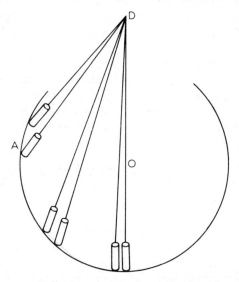

Fig. 1.15 In the graded differential orientation model all receptors are in line with an
anterior point D. Again, these are supposed to be neighbouring receptors and the scale has
been purposely distorted. O is the occular centre (cf. Fig. 1.6.). (From Laties and Enoch,
1971. © 1971 The C. V. Mosby Co., St Louis.)

While the Stiles–Crawford effect is well authenticated on a macro-scale,
directional effects are hard to analyse in individual receptors even though
observations on isolated receptors have yielded valuable insight into their
properties (p. 139). The reason is that, with a diameter of 1–2 μ, they cannot be
fruitfully studied with simple geometrical optics, and the more demanding
approach based on diffraction theory is, at present, hampered by our ignorance of
the details of refractive index variations in the sundry receptor components
(Fig. 1.17). Receptors can be imagined to act like wave-guides, a special property

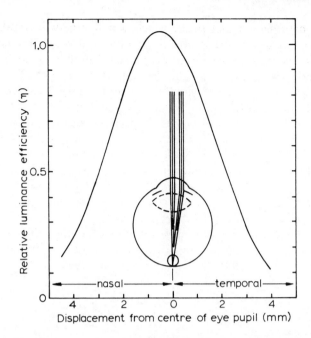

Displacement from centre of eye pupil (mm)

Fig. 1.16 The so-called retinal direction effect. Given two equally intense pencils of light, one of which enters the eye through the pupillary centre, but the other through the periphery at various distances in turn (abscissa), the luminous efficiency of the latter can be determined in terms of the former (ordinate). (From Weale, 1968a. © Oliver & Boyd, Edinburgh and London.)

of which is that, in certain circumstances, a significant fraction of the energy can be pictured to travel outside their geometrical confines: their effective cross-sectional area is, therefore, greater than their actual one, and the consequences which this may have for interaction between tightly-packed receptors are not yet fully known.

The microscopic structure of photo-receptors has been known for almost a century (Fig. 1.18). Their outer limb or segment is where energy acts. It is attached by means of a cilium (Fig. 1.19) to a twin structure, the ellipsoid and myoid, known together as the inner limb. The large concentration of mitochrondria in the ellipsoid stresses its metabolic importance. In the cones of birds and lower vertebrates, this part may contain an oil droplet with varying absorption characteristics: it may act as a light filter perhaps as part of a mechanism for colour vision. The rod is connected to its nucleus by a fibre, and then terminates in a spherule. By contrast, the cone nucleus adjoins the inner limb and has a short connection to a pedicle. Both units then meet a synapse, a morphological discontinuity found throughout the central nervous system. Ultra-microscopic studies reveal special areas of high electron density in synaptic regions: they are thought to provide the bridge-head for the transmission of responses to subsequent stages (cf. p. 32).

First some consideration has to be given to the ultra-structure of the outer limbs. At first sight, both rods and cones appear to share a similar composition

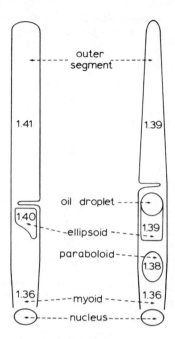

Fig. 1.17   The parts of a rod (left) and a cone (right) with 'average' refractive indices. (From Weale, 1968b. © North-Holland Publishing Co. Amsterdam, 1968.)

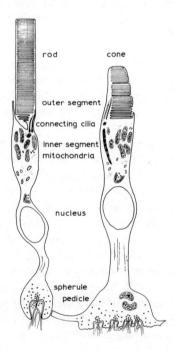

Fig. 1.18   Schematic diagram of rod and cone cells of the mammalian retina based on electron microscopic observations. (From Ripps and Weale, 1976. © Academic Press Inc. New York & London.)

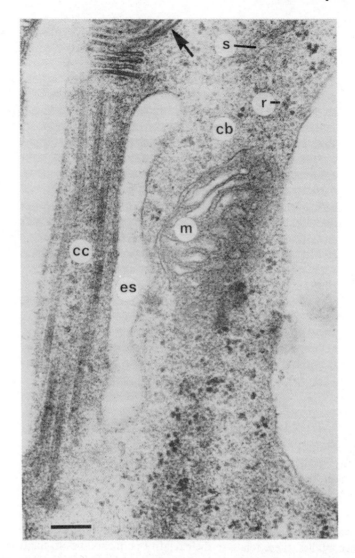

Fig. 1.19 Longitudinal section through a rat rod showing both the connecting cilium (cc) and the cytoplasmic bridge (cb), separated by a channel of extracellular space (es). Ribosomes (r), saccules (s) and mitochondria (m) have direct access to the disc membranes (arrow) through the cytoplasmic bridge. Bar = 200 nm. (After Richardson, 1969.)

made up of lamellae (Fig. 1.20), many hundreds of which are found in each outer limb. One fundamental difference is indicated: the rod lamellae are contained in a sac – the plasma membrane – from which they are separated. But the lamellae of the cones are onè continuous sheet of plasma membrane, formed by in-folding. The cone disks are 14 nm, the rod disks 18 nm, in thickness (Dowling, 1967). It is this lamination that is responsible for the birefringence of rods and cones.

However, though ultra-structurally there appears to be lamellar uniformity, Kaplan *et al.*, (1978) point to a birefringence gradient along the rod axis.

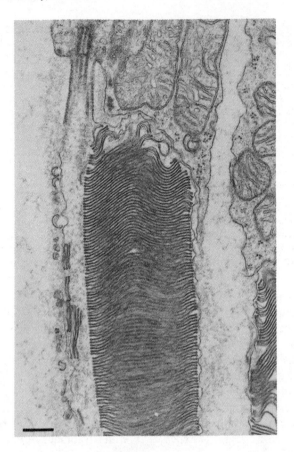

Fig. 1.20a   Proximal part of the rod. (Note cilium top left; cf. Fig. 1.19). Rod lamellae are formed near the top. Bar = 500 nm. (Original: courtesy J. Marshall, Institute of Ophthalmology.)

Moreover, clear distinctions between rods and cones are revealed by birefringence studies: these relate to their relative permeabilities to fixatives such as formaldehyde and glutaraldehyde. This method has also been used in histochemical studies which confirm Weale's prediction (1971) that rod birefringence is due to more than one stratified component. In a study of frog rods, it was shown that anisotropy extends to acidic polysaccharides and free aldehyde groups (perhaps artifactually generated by formalin fixative) and the oligosaccharide chains of the light-sensitive pigment rhodopsin. The poly- and oligo-saccharide orientation is connected with the preferential orientations of photo-pigment, molecules with their dipoles parallel to the planes of the lamellae, a feature which lends significance to the axial inclination of the receptors in various parts of the eye (p. 20). Although the light-absorbing pigment molecules are therefore constrained in planes perpendicular to the receptor axis (Kawamura et al., 1977), they are free to rotate in those planes (Brownian movement) as can be demonstrated e.g. if glutaraldehyde immobilizes them before they have been

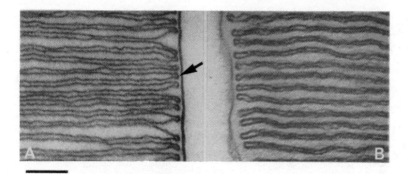

Fig. 1.20b Longitudinal section of portions of outer segments of rod (A) and cone (B) from the same preparation of monkey retina. The rods consistently exhibit a wider intradisc space as compared with the cones, and also demonstrate a characteristic button-like ending at the edge of the disc (arrow). Bar = 0.1 μ (From Dowling, 1967. © 1967 by John M. Allen. Reprinted by permission of Harper & Row, Publishers, Inc.)

photolyzed with plane polarized light, and, the plane of polarization having been turned through 90°, extinction can be demonstrated. This is impossible in the absence of the paralyzing fixative, as Brownian movement destroys the dichroism produced by the first light exposure.

In fact, the relation between the visual pigment molecule and the membrane is nothing like as simple as one surmises if the former is imagined to be a smooth elongated body, and the latter bounded by two comparatively large surfaces. If X-rays are passed through outer segments of known orientation, it is possible to detect diffraction patterns akin to those associated with crystals largely as a result of the work of the Braggs. The rhodopsin, while in contact with some 20 per cent of the membrane fatty acids at any one instant, extends evenly across each segment but protrudes through the membrane: its polypeptide chain may cut it at least five times (Dratz *et al.*, 1979) which is why earlier workers believed the molecules to reside in the surface. Contact with the lipid layer is important from the point of view of the stabilization of the rhodopsin molecule within the saccule.

Visual pigments

The visual pigments – as the transducing pigments found in receptor outer limbs are collectively referred to on account of their function and nature – have been known for just over a century. They are chromoproteins, the spectral properties of which are determined largely by a retinene chain (Fig. 1.21). The unexposed pigment present as about 50 per cent of the dry weight of the lamellae, exists in the 11-cis form, its stereo-complexion changing to all-trans as a result of the absorption of a quantum of radiation. Green *et al.* (1977) have shown that the resultant isomerization of the rhodopsin molecule occurs within less than 9 pico-seconds and that the half-time occupies some 3 ps. X-ray diffraction from bleached and unbleached retinae shows significant structural changes in the disk membranes and furthermore locates at least part of the pigment molecule in the cytoplasmic membrane: the pigment is probably embedded only in one side of the

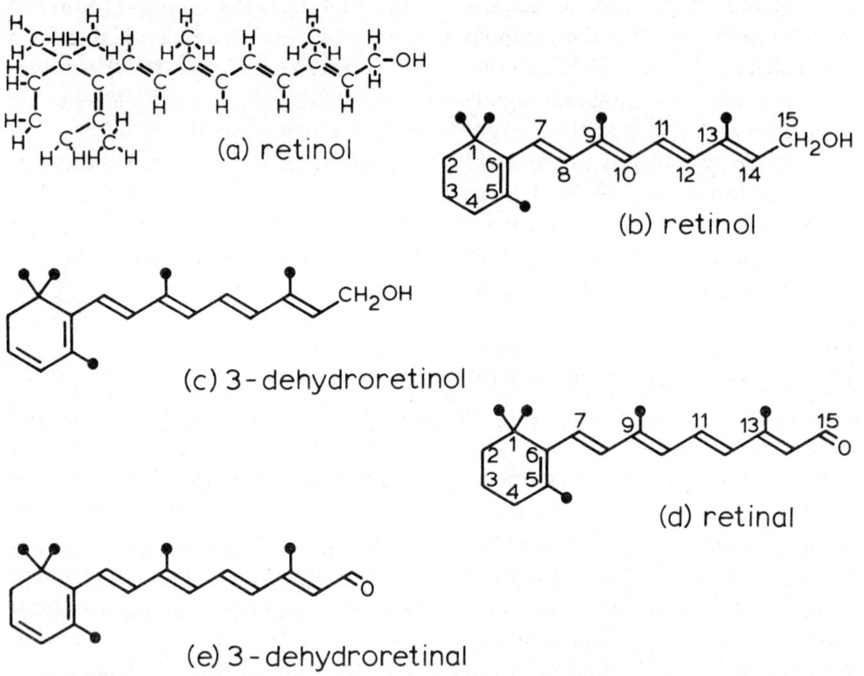

(a) retinol

(b) retinol

(c) 3-dehydroretinol

(d) retinal

(e) 3-dehydroretinal

Fig. 1.21   Structural formulae for compounds related to retinal. (a) Complete structure of retinol; (b) abbreviated formula for retinol, showing the numbering of the atoms of the carbon skeleton; (c) 3-dehydroretinol; (d) retinal; (e) 3-dehydroretinal. (From Knowles and Dartnall, 1977. © Academic Press Inc. New York & London, 1977.)

bi-layer as it has been shown to abut an aqueous interface, and to be asymmetrically placed in the membrane (Dratz *et al.* 1972).

Being such an important structural component of the rod lamellae, the pigment partakes of their continuous assembly and ultimate disposal by the phagocytic processes of the pigment epithelium that envelop the apices of the rods (Hall *et al.*, 1969). As mentioned in more detail in Ch. 2, the situation differs in the cones where the apicopetal displacement of the lamellae is replaced by molecular turnover, because the cone outer limb consists of a single sheet (cf. p. 25).

Vertebrate visual pigments share certain properties even though not all of them have been found to be significant for the initiation of the visual response. They all absorb radiations of wavelengths in or near the 'visible' part of the electromagnetic spectrum. There is no action without absorption. Their quantum efficiency γ (number of molecules photolysed per number of quanta absorbed) is unity or just below. Their extinction coefficient is near a theoretical maximum based on the effective cross-section of a hydrogen molecule. In general, as we have already noted, their steric (spatial) configuration changes following the capture of a quantum. This leads to a change in their spectral absorption, and to a sequence of 'dark' reactions, so called because they are revealed in the absence of irradiation, even though they may occur in its presence. They give rise to products of varying life-times. The stoichiometric balance of the 'photo-products' varies with pH and temperature: in fact, some of the life-times are so short at room and body temperatures that the compounds can be obtained in an identifiable form only when cooled to $-90\,°C$ or even $-180\,°C$ (Kawamura *et al.*, 1977). Another important, and physiologically significant feature is that photolysed pigments can regenerate and return to their virgin form. In the living eye, this is achieved by darkness. When we stay in the dark, our visual pigments reach their maximum concentration (cf. pp. 59, 70, 91). Azuma *et al.* (1977) showed (on perfused frog retinae) that rhodopsin can regenerate almost fully – even in the absence of the pigment epithelium the contiguity between the rods and which used to be thought essential. One proviso, however, was that the light exposure preceding regeneration should not have been excessive. This study reveals important differences between frog rhodopsin regeneration and the type claimed to exist in man by Campbell and Rushton in 1955: but this may be due to inadequacies in the latter study as the agreement with the data due to Weale and, later, Alpern and Pugh is much better.

The detailed properties of visual pigments have, however, been studied in extracts obtained from the dark-adapted retinae of many species notably frogs, cattle, rats, and sundry fish. Although we stressed above that there is no photic action without absorption, the latter has to be inferred from measurements of intensities of monochromatic radiation that has traversed pigment solutions without being absorbed. The ratio of the transmitted intensities to the incident ones $I(T) \div I(I)$ is the spectral transmissivity $T(\lambda)$, where λ is the wavelength. We define the density $D(\lambda)$ as

$$D(\lambda) = -\log_{10} T(\lambda) = \alpha(\lambda)cx$$

where $\alpha(\lambda)$ is the extinction coefficient, c the concentration, and x the path length of the pigment complex: the latter may be the length of a photo-receptor outer limb e.g. in the studies mentioned in the previous paragraph. The absorption $A(\lambda)$ being given by $A(\lambda) + T(\lambda) = 1$, if reflection losses are allowed for, it follows that

$$A(\lambda) = 1 - \exp(-.4343)\alpha(\lambda)cx$$

which reduces to $A(\lambda) = .4343\alpha(\lambda)cx$ if the term on the RHS is small. This tells us that, under these conditions, the absorption is nearly $D(\lambda) \div 2.3$. Modern photo-electron multiplier radiometers enable one to measure D without appreciably changing c in the above equation. The reason is that their great sensitivity allows the use of extremely feeble incident intensities $I(I)$.

It can be shown on the basis of a number of simplifying assumptions that the relation between photolysing intensity I (P, λ), exposure time t, and pigment concentration $c(I, t)$ is given by

$$c(I, t) = c(0)\exp\left[-\alpha(\lambda)\gamma I(P, \lambda)t\right]$$

where $c(0)$ represents the concentration prior to exposure. $\alpha(\lambda)\gamma$ is called the photo-sensitivity: in SI units it is of the order of 10^{17}: it is the reciprocal of that irradiance $I(P, \lambda)$ t which reduces the concentration to $1/e$ of its original value. If we determine this value with radiations of different wavelengths we establish the spectral variation of the relation

$$\alpha(\lambda)I(P, \lambda)t = \text{constant}$$

as γ is in principle invariable. If t is kept constant and $I(P,\lambda)$ is defined as $1/S(\lambda)$ we see that

$$S(\lambda) \propto \alpha(\lambda)$$

In other words, the spectral sensitivity of the pigment, and therefore that of the receptor containing it, is proportional to the pigment extinction coefficient (Fig. 1.22). It is one of the triumphs and disasters of visual science that this relation holds e.g. for the extinction coefficient of human rhodopsin, the rod pigment, and the human rod sensitivity curve. It is a triumph because the relation seems simple only in retrospect, and a disaster because it has led to a large number of analogous exercises of curve-fitting in circumstances based on very different premises: as such it has led to many unnecessary misunderstandings (cf. Ch. 2).

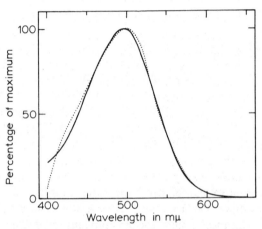

Fig. 1.22 ———————— Density spectrum of human visual purple. • • • • • • • • • • Spectral sensitivity of dark-adapted extra-foveal region. (After Crescitelli and Dartnall, 1953.)

The human rod pigment rhodopsin or visual purple consists of the aldehyde of retinol (vitamin A_1) and a protein called opsin. The former compound, known as 11-cis retinal is the light absorbing moiety of the molecule the weight of which is $\sim 40\,000$ (cf. Ostroy, 1977). Its concentration in human rods is 0.1 mM, which is high as compared with bovine (0.06 mM), but low in comparison with frog (2 mM) values: thus, with up to 1000 disks (p. 24) the number of molecules per human outer limb is approximately ten million: in 1942 Hecht, Shlaer and Pirenne pointed out that a rod can be stimulated with but one of these molecules absorbing a quantum, although more than one rod may have to be stimulated for a perception of light to be generated.

The link between 11-cis retinal on the one hand and the protein and the associated lipid on the other alters following the absorption of a quantum. The Schiff base binding site ($-C{=}N-$) is involved in an early dark-reaction in a deprotonation and subsequently in a protonation: the former occurs when the short-lived product of photolysis metarhodopsin I changes to the long-lived metarhodopsin II, the latter when meta II is converted into meta III (cf. Table 1.1).

Table 1.1   Human rhodopsin reactions following exposure to light.

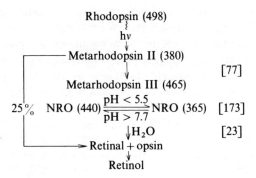

Honig *et al.* (1976) have stressed that photolysis may not lead simply to an alteration in the Schiff base but also to a reorientation of the chromophore, i.e. the retinal. It is worth noting that no such significant steric change is likely to take place before the formation of metarhodopsin III: when single frog rods are examined spectroscopically and dark-reactions are recorded with plane-polarized light, it can be shown that the sign of the outer segment dichroism does not alter till the retinol (vitamin A) stage is reached. The kinetics of these transformations depend on a variety of factors, and the figures in round brackets refer to the wavelength maximum (nm) of the extinction spectrum, those in square brackets to the half-times of the reactions (secs). This relatively simple sequence can be detected at human body temperature: the equilibrium between the two forms of N-retinylidene opsin (NRO) is biased towards the NRO (365) form. The shunt on the left (Brin and Ripps, 1977) may play a role in the regeneration of rhodopsin, but as the full significance of dark reactions remains to be elucidated, there is no point in speculating on the reason for this pecularity.

We shall see in a moment that the rapid cis-trans change in the polyene chain of the chromophore (p. 26) occurs long before a physiological rod response can be detected, and it would, of course, be surprising if as complicated a structure as the receptor outer limb could respond to an unamplified physically minimal stimulus. One reason for this is that, in the detection of a visual signal and, therefore, in the prior generation of a visual response, the signal-to-noise ratio must assume a significant value, usually taken as three. Ashmore and Falk (1977) have confirmed (in a study of the retina of the dogfish) that photon noise has a large inverse temperature dependence: but at 37°C, it would correspond to one isomerization every 30 s per human rod. This is an acceptably low figure.

Part of the explanation of this is to be found in the good protection of the binding site (p. 28) linking chromophore and protein, namely a protonated Schiff base bond which can be exposed by the hydrogenation of rhodopsin irradiated in the presence of sodium borohydride. While the early 'dark' changes, e.g. MR I → MR II (Table1.1) involve major conformational changes, binding sites appear to be freed only when this reaction is complete. The thermal decay of MR II leads to a separation of retinal from opsin; during the change MR II → MR III a number of sulphydryl groups are exposed probably as a result of this opening up of the molecule, likened by Dartnall to a lock-and-key situation.

Electrical responses to illumination

It has been known for well over a century that the illumination of the intact human eye leads to changes in electrical potential e.g. if one (active) electrode is made to abut the cornea and another (indifferent one) adheres to the forehead. The changes are complex, being made up of potentials generated in the receptors, the neural retina, and the pigment epithelium out of phase in relation to one another, and varying in specifically different ways with such parameters as stimulus intensity, level of adaptation, stimulus duration etc. The potential complex is referred to as the electro-retinogram or ERG, (Fig. 1.23a). Its earliest component, the negative late a-receptor component is associated with receptor function. It can be isolated from all other retinal potentials by retinal perfusion with sodium aspartate in a concentration as low as 10 mM. The later positive b-component originates more centrally: it is accompanied by a d.c. component, also positive, which has much the same duration as the stimulus that produces the ERG. The last slow positive excursion or component is derived from the pigment epithelium. In some animals such as the frog, an off-effect due to stimulus cessation can also be observed. The ERG has a diagnostic value, pioneered as a tool for this purpose by the Swedish ophthalmologist Karpe.

In recent years the ERG has been much refined, and used as a valuable research method throwing light on the above relation between the sequence of post-photolytic changes in the molecule on the one hand and the initiation of the visual response on the other. Improved stimulus control and electrode technology have made it possible to isolate two important potentials preceding the a− wave. Collectively known as the early receptor potential (ERP), they are referred to as RI and RII. The amplitude of RI can be used within certain limits as a counter of quanta and of bleached photo-pigment molecules. Moreover, the timing of R_1 ((Fig. 1.23b) all but coincides with the onset of the formation of MR II (cf. Table 1.1) whereas that of R_2 is three or four times as slow. While the association between R_1 and pigment molecules is strong, it is still open to argument (Ostroy, 1977). Galloway (1967) has shown that the ERP can be recorded in man, and Goldstein and Berson (1970) have used it for diagnostic purposes.

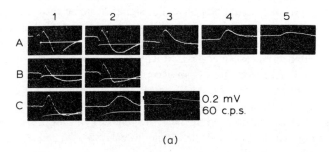

(a)

Fig. 1.23a Electroretinogram (ERG) with different intensities and/or rise times of white light stimuli shown in the lower of each pair of traces. The numbers (1 5) refer to decreasing intensities. Rise times: A = 25 milliseconds, B = 100 milliseconds, C = 230 milliseconds. (From Bornschein and Gunkel, 1956. © Ophthalmic Publishing Co. Chicago.)

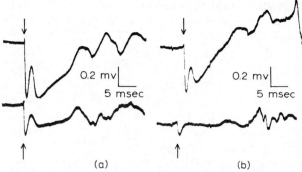

(a)   (b)

Fig. 1.23b (a) Upper trace: Early receptor potential (ERP) obtained with a single flash with eye adapted to room lighting. Lower trace: second flash one minute later. (b) Upper trace: single flash after 20 minutes' dark adaptation. Lower trace: single flash 30 seconds later, showing very small ERP. (From Galloway, 1967. © 1967 *British Journal of Ophthalmology*.)

R_2 is a harder element to tackle. Its behaviour under the action of formaldehyde and at high temperatures has led to the suggestion that it is contingent on the intactness of the lamellar structure of the rod. Unlike another fixative, namely glutaraldehyde, which abolishes R_2 and alters drastically that part of birefringence which is due to the arrangement of molecules rather than to their structure, formaldehyde has little, or slowly acting, influence on either property. Again, R_2 is abolished and birefringence materially changed (in frog rods) at a temperature somewhat lower than that at which the denaturation of rhodopsin vitiates photo-stimulation (Fig. 1.24). Thus the structure of the rod membrane and the saccules is irreversibly altered at 51° C whereas about 60° C

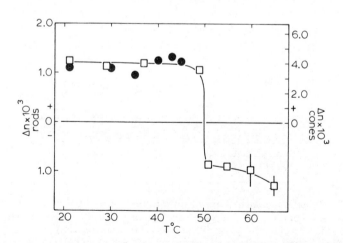

Fig. 1.24 The effect of thermal shock on the birefringence of frog rods (□) and cones (●). No cone was detectable in the microscopic field above a temperature of 45°. Rods elongated drastically at 51° C (at a temperature lower than that needed to denature rhodopsin, i.e. 61°) and their birefringence changed irreversibly from positive to negative. (After Weale, 1971.)

are needed to render a rhodopsin molecule unphotolysable because heat has 'denatured' it. And while we are on structural changes, it may also be noted that exposure to light leads to a small reduction in the size of the outer limb. This was first suggested by Weale on the basis of birefringence changes, confirmed on the basis of bleaching energetics by Falk and Fatt, and supported also by an X-ray diffraction study of isolated frog retinae by Chabre and Cavaggioni. The decrease amounts to between one part in 10^4 to one in 10^3 and cannot, of course, be observed directly under the microscope. Such a configurational change – conceivably due to one in inter-lamellar spacing could be accompanied by a charge displacement leading to the generation of R_2.

How light-absorption by rhodopsin leads to the ionic changes needed to produce a propagatable potential in the receptor outer limb is still uncertain, but the ideas on this have been clarified largely as a result of the work done by Hagins and his colleagues. Using a triple electrode, with the tips laterally separated by 0.1 mm, and one of them lagging by a similar distance behind the other two, Hagins *et al.* (1970) measured the radial resistivity of thin strips of rat retina, chosen because it contains almost only rods. The resistivity equalled that of the surrounding extra-cellular fluid in the neighbourhood of the outer and inner limbs, but rose toward the synaptic region (p. 21): here the space not occupied by receptors is filled by parts of Müller cells which are glial structures, radially spanning the retina.

Using the triple micro-electrodes the above authors determined the photo-voltaic changes along the receptor layer. Together with the resistance data, the latter yielded the transmembrane current due to illumination (flash intensities of 2×10^{10} and $8 \times 10^{10} q/cm^2$) as a function of position along the receptor (Fig. 1.25). Illuminated parts gave rise to a positive current: the outer segment then

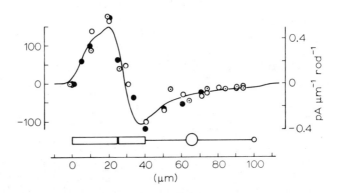

Fig. 1.25   Radial component $D(x)$ of divergence of interstitial current in uniformly illuminated slices of rat retina. The points show peak values of $D(x)$ for slices illuminated with 560 nm flashes of intensity 2×10^{10} photons cm^{-2} (filled circles) or 8×10^{10} photons cm^{-2} (open and dotted circles). All responses are scaled to amplitudes that would have been obtained for saturating flashes ($> 2 \times 10^{11}$ photons cm^{-2}). The curve is the theoretical value of $D(x)$ expected from a layer of model rods assuming that the membrane drive current is distributed uniformly along the outer segments of the rods, and the recordings are made with a triplet of micro-electrodes with radial intertip spacings of $10 \mu m$. (From *The Vertebrate Retina: Principles of Structure and Function* by R. W. Rodieck. W. H. Freeman and Company. © 1973)

acts in this condition as a source. Unilluminated parts and the rest of the photo-receptor act as a sink. It was also shown that rods possess an extra-cellular current of strength 71 pA opposed to the photo-current, and present in the dark. It leads to the synaptic region being at a potential positive with respect to the outer limb apex.

Light reduces the dark current – for which the outer limb acts as a sink – and the spatial distribution of which mirrors that of the photo-current: this suggests that the two currents flow through the same ionic channels in the plasma-membrane. Light reduces the ionic conductance: according to Arden and Ernst (1970), insofar as pigeon cones are concerned, Na^+ is the only ion that needs considering.

As illumination, moreover, hyperpolarizes both rods and cones, a per-meability change must be involved, which may be the fundamental event to occur. Thus Arden and Ernst believe that the membrane potential of cones is governed by the distribution of anions in illumination, but by an increase in cations in darkness. Yoshikami and Hagins (1971) have suggested that calcium provides an ionic plug and is released as a result of a conformational change in rhodopsin molecules (p. 29) following the absorption of radiation. On illumi-nation this internal transmitter closes channels that are permeable to sodium ions, which carry the 'dark' photo-current. This is reduced in lizard cones both by Ca and by light. As there is some doubt whether the amount of Ca^{2+} freed is adequate to the task (see below) other ionic candidates have been looked for. Bellhorn and Lewis's discovery in 1976 of special concentrates of Ba^{2+} in the photo-receptors of cats (partly paralleling that of calcium) has prompted Brown and Flaming to study the effects of these two ions on perfused isolated retinae of the toad *Bufo marinus*. Insofar as barium had effects opposite to those produced by calcium on the photic responses recorded intracellularly from the rod outer segment, it mimicked the effects of dark-adaptation, i.e. the opposite of the light-adaptational parallel of calcium. Arden (1977) has stressed that more than one photo-induced voltage has to be postulated so that the behaviour of rat rods may be accounted for. The Ca hypothesis is easier to test in cones which may be without intracellular spaces by virtue of the manner in which their plasma membrane is folded (cf. p. 25). This means that there is no need to *infer* the ion concentration as is necessary for the closed saccules of rods. Arden and Low (1978) calculate that the effective availability of calcium is too low to allow this ion to act as sole internal transmitter: an unspecified molecule, made available in the membrane following quantal absorption, is also needed. These and other considerations intensified the search for other candidates to act in the transmis-sion process. A photically activated phosphodiasterase was discovered in the outer segments of rods: it catalyses the hydrolysis of cyclic guanosine monophosphate, or cGMP. In other neurones, cyclic nucleotides are co-factors for a kinase ultimately controlling membrane permeability, and the idea of cGMP acting in a similar way finds tentative support from the observation that the permeability of the rod outer limbs and the concentration of cGMP are correlated in a variety of conditions.

This crude outline of receptor studies must suffice to indicate that, while great strides are being made in our understanding of the formation of a graded potential in the photo-receptor, it is still incomplete. It is noteworthy, e.g. that

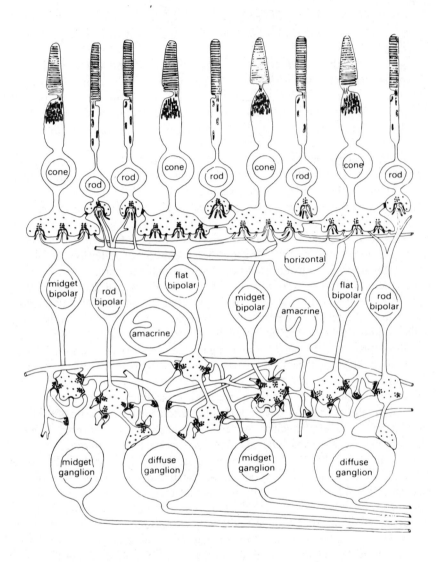

Fig. 1.26 A synthetic diagram of neural contacts in the retina. (After Dowling and Boycott, 1966.)

the sensitivity of the rod to light – which, after all, measures its functional performance – is independent of the external Ca^{2+} concentration within wide limits. The restoration of the sensitivity, and the extent to which this may or may not be tied to the regeneration of photolysed pigment (Brin and Ripps, 1977) is also a wide open question.

The inner retinal layers

The next section of the vertebrate retina shows much greater inter-species variation than is true of the bacillary (i.e. photo-receptor) layer. From an evolutionary point of view this cannot occasion surprise. To a first approximation, visual pigment absorption spectra reflect the product of the spectral distribution of low (daylight) and high (moonlight) colour temperatures respectively and the spectral transmissivity of the extra-ocular environment. In the case of aquatic species, this can vary considerably. Grafted on to this principal division, there is the sub-set of different cones, providing the potential for colour vision. There are further refinements, e.g. the distribution of receptors on either side of the projection on the retina of the horizon, but these merely elaborate the fundamental principle that the most economic use of radiation occurs when the difference between the emission spectrum of the illuminant as measured at the retina and the absorption spectrum of the transducer is a minimum. When overlap between the two is negligible, radiation fails to act. This is why we cannot see radio-waves.

However, in the next, the inner nuclear, layer (Fig. 1.26), there exist inter-cellular paths and ramifications, demonstrably of use in information processing. And as the photic information content reaching most eyes is too great for comfort, this weeding out of data uninteresting to the individual cannot begin too soon. If we make a number of simplifying assumptions, we find that the number of optical degrees of freedom is equal to the number of receptors, e.g. in the human retina and especially in its less peripheral parts. An optical degree of freedom (d.o.f.) may be represented by the smallest areal element in an image for which an intensity value has to be available if the object which it represents is to be completely defined. Thus diffraction makes it unnecessary to specify the flux at an infinity of vanishingly small points. The optics of the eye yield a value of approximately 0.15 d.o.f./μ sq (Fig. 1.27) and this is of the same order as the receptor density. But if every receptor had an optic nerve fibre of its own, severe anatomical problems would ensue. In man, the ratio of receptor to fibre is roughly 100:1, and the decimation of information which this necessitates is carried out in part in the bipolar layer.

At this stage we may note that the nucleus (soma) of the generalized cell receives afferent information via dendrites and transmits it via its single efferent axon.

Fig. 1.26 offers a schematic survey of the organization of the primate retina, and indicates that the rod spherules and cone pedicles synapse with different types of bipolar cell. Rods connect with mop, cones with midget and flat, bipolar cells (Dowling and Boycott, 1966). In the central part of the retina, midget bipolars synapse with only one cone pedicle bar but do so in more than one place. Kolb (1970) has suggested that there are, in fact, two midget bipolar cells per cone, and Missotten (1974) puts the ratio as high as 3 to 1. Flat bipolar cells, on the other hand, connect with several cones via superficial contact at the pedicles. Together with the horizontal and amacrine cells, the bipolars form the inner nuclear layer. Horizontal cells appear to fulfil a transverse interactive function: they link 7–12 receptors via their bases, perhaps providing a pathway for feed-back responses in the outer synaptic (plexiform) layer. Wässle et al. (1978) have

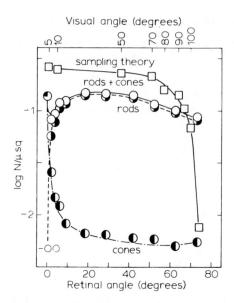

Fig. 1.27   To show that the number of receptors per unit area as a function of retinal locus (abscissa) closely parallels the theoretically largest useful number of sampling points needed to define an image (cf. Fig. 1.9). (From Weale, 1976. © 1976 Optical Society of America.)

quantitatively studied whole-mount preparations of cat retinae. They Azan-stained them so that the cone inner segments and nuclei could be clearly distinguished from the rods, and determined what contact the dendritic trees of horizontal A and B cells made with the cones (A-cells which, unlike the B-type have no axon, have the larger dendritic field of the two). A plot of the population density of cones (solid line) as a function of distance from the area centralis is shown in Fig. 1.28. The broken line represents 75 per cent of the values shown by the continuous one, and it is clear that both the A cells (o) and the B-cells (●) contact over 75 per cent of the cone population per sq mm.

The dendrites of amacrine cells perhaps fulfil an analogous function in the inner plexiform layer: here they interact not only with other amacrine dendrites but also with the synaptic terminals of bipolar cells, and almost always with dendrites and even the soma of the ganglion cells. The latter are large cells with long axons which form the fibres of the optic nerve. In the cat retina, rod bipolar cells synapse on two types of amacrine cell, and cone bipolars connect directly with only one of the types and with ganglion cells. It has been suggested that these morphological differences may have correlates in the organization of the receptive field (cf. p. 41), and that may be related to rod-dominated retinae though not everyone is agreed that the cat retina is typical in this respect.

Rohen and Mrodzinsky (1955) have shown that, in the rat retina, the volumes of the retinal nuclei significantly increase following prolonged illumination to a 200 w source at a distance of 50 cm (Fig. 1.29). It is noteworthy that this occurs earliest in the ganglion and last in the receptor layer in broad keeping with the notion of convergence.

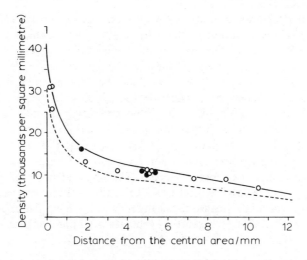

Fig. 1.28 Comparison of the cone density and the density of terminal aggregations of both types of horizontal cell along a retinal strip. (From Wässle, Boycott and Peichl, 1978. © The Royal Society, London.)

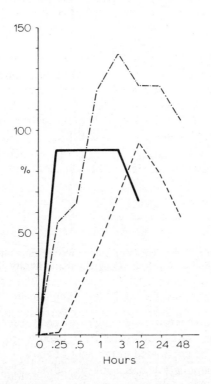

Fig. 1.29 Representation of percentage volume changes as a function of duration of illumination (intensity: 200 w): ———— ganglion cells, — · — · — . inner nuclear layer, — — — — — outer nuclear layer. (After Rohen and Mrodzinsky, 1955.)

The numerical evaluation of cell distribution, and especially of their contacts (cf. Kolb, 1970), is no simple matter. Although various techniques are available for the identification of the above and other cells, staining gives only a minimum density, and, if specific, may miss some types altogether. Shrinkage is a problem bedevilling all histology and there are those who claim that it may introduce errors as large as 20 per cent. Nevertheless, excellent quantitative work has been done on the retina during this century: understandably the data on primates in general, and on man in particular, are sparse. A quantitative comparison of the densities of rods and cones on the one hand, and ganglion cells on the other reveals interesting features (Fig. 1.30). Except in the para-foveal regions, the receptors are much the more numerous. The preponderance of ganglion and other cells, just outside the central area is to be attributed to their expulsion from the foveal centre either because classically they (and the bipolar cells) would lead to a deterioration of vision because they might scatter light, or because the retinal

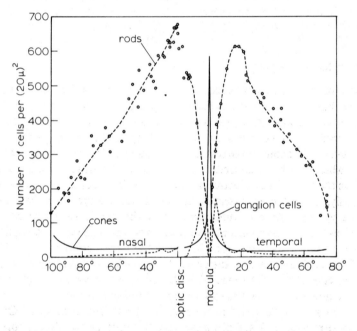

Fig. 1.30 Comparison of the density of human retinal ganglion cells in the horizontal meridian in a square having a side 20 μ in length with the density of rods and cones. (After Oppel, 1967.)

blood supply in this area is too inadequate to provide them with metabolites. This perturbation in what would otherwise be a smooth angular function of cell distribution should be considered in the light of a study on the distribution of retinal elements in mammals such as monkeys and cats, where cones and ganglion cells form mosaics. The advantage of regular over random patterns is that the former eliminate 'holes' which demand high cell densities or wider arborisation. If monkey cones were distributed randomly (in the presence of rods), midget bipolars might find it hard to home onto a cone, so increasing the expenditure of evolutionary or developmental energy. The disturbance of ganglionic regularity near the fovea may help to explain why this region is poorer in summating sub-threshold impulses than is true of the more peripheral regions.

The diminution of visual acuity with distance from the fovea is clearly not attributable to the variation of cone density so much as to that of ganglion cells which receive information from cones. Frisén and Frisén (1976) have shown in a painstaking study that there is a close linear relation between the distance between ganglion cells and the spatial wavelength resolved in the relevant part of the retina respectively. This illustrates the importance of the notion of the final common path: while resolution depends on the density of neurones connecting with the cerebral cortex, it is to be noted that the convergence ratio is large in the retinal periphery (p. 15) but drops to about unity, its optimum, in the retinal centre. However, we shall note below that this type of comparison involves a gross, if convenient, simplification: cells are not characterized only by their population density but mainly by their orbits of activity, and, in the case of primates, it may be best to elaborate this point when we have reached the discussion of the cortex (p. 45).

The path to the cortex

The axons of the ganglion cells run along the vitreal side of the retina toward the optic disk, known functionally as the blind spot. It was discovered by the French scientist Mariotte who greatly pleased his monarch by imaging in turn the heads of a number of his courtiers on the royal optic disk so creating transient decapitations. The axons of the central retinal ganglion cells follow typical arcs to the disk which can be visualized as the blue arcs of Purkyně when red light is flashed on the fovea. The collective of fibres leave the eye at the optic disk, where, incidentally, major blood vessels of the retinal vasculature (cf. p. 98) enter and leave the eye-ball. At this vulnerable point the eye is strengthened by the collagenous lamina cribrosa, a net-work of fibrils through which the optic nerve fibres penetrate to leave the bony orbit via the optic foramen (Fig. 1.31). The nerves from both eyes meet at the optic chiasma where 70 per cent cross over to the contra-lateral side of the head while the remainder stay on the ipsilateral side. The reassembled nerve bundles travel to the lateral geniculate body (Fig. 1.32a), a layered relay station, the function of which is still not fully understood. Of the six layers, those numbered 1, 4, 6 counting from the inner aspect contain fibres from the contra lateral eye, while layers 2, 3, and 5 consist of those of the ipsi-lateral axons. The fibres synapse in the lateral geniculate nucleus with the more numerous optic radiations which lead to Brodmann's area 17 in the occipital part of the cortex.

It is clear from Fig. 1.32b that the left lateral geniculate body receives an input from fibres stimulated by the right visual field which is projected onto the left retinal halves and *vice versa*. But just because the striate area of the cortex is frequently looked on as 'the brain' insofar as vision is concerned, it would be erroneous to see in it something final. In a sense, it is also a relay station. In some frontally-eyed animals, such as the cat, the input for the two eyes is partly combined at the most peripherally possible point, namely the lateral geniculate body. In man and other primates, on the other hand, this combination takes place

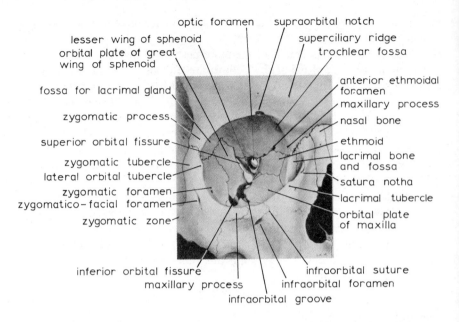

optic foramen
supraorbital notch
lesser wing of sphenoid
superciliary ridge
orbital plate of great
trochlear fossa
wing of sphenoid
anterior ethmoidal
fossa for lacrimal gland
foramen
maxillary process
zygomatic process
nasal bone
superior orbital fissure
ethmoid
zygomatic tubercle
lacrimal bone
and fossa
lateral orbital tubercle
zygomatic foramen
satura notha
zygomatico-facial foramen
lacrimal tubercle
zygomatic zone
orbital plate
of maxilla

inferior orbital fissure
infraorbital suture
maxillary process
infraorbital foramen
infraorbital groove

Fig. 1.31   The right orbit viewed along its axis. (From Warwick (ed.), 1976. © 1976 H. K. Lewis & Co., London.)

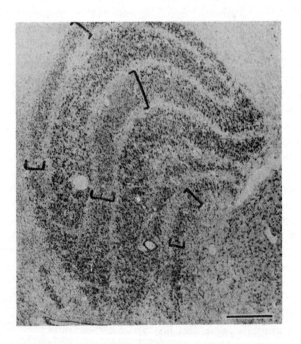

Fig. 1.32a   Transverse section of the lateral geniculate nucleus of a macaque monkey showing localised cell atrophy in three laminæ, following a macular lesion in the retina of the opposite side. The numbering of the layers is from right to left, i.e. degeneration has occurred in the 1st, 4th and 6th layers. Bar = 0.5 mm. (After Le Gros Clark, 1949.)

R   L

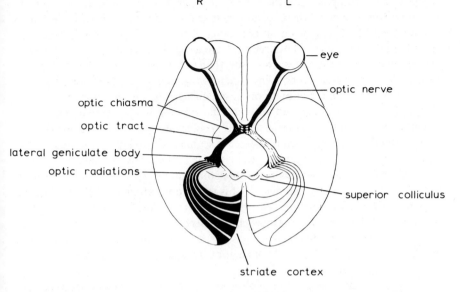

Fig. 1.32b   Diagram of the retino-geniculo-cortical pathway in a higher mammal. The brain is viewed from below. The right half of each retina, shown in black, projects to the right hemisphere (to the left, in the figure since it is viewed from below): thus the right hemisphere receives an input from both eyes and is concerned with the left half-field of vision. (After Hubel and Wiesel, 1977.)

in one of the six layers of the striate cortex, as we shall note below. Axons from this area follow paths to a variety of stations, and also return to the lateral geniculate body, which, in turn, sends centrifugal fibres to the retina: in the parlance of communications theory, they probably carry feed-back information.

This cortico-geniculate feed-back has to be borne in mind in connection with the demonstration that some units in the normal cat's lateral geniculate body are weakly sensitive to orientation. 'Weakly' means in this context that the polar diagram has a length-to-width ratio of 2 or less, and Daniels *et al.* (1977) have shown indirectly that a retinal projection is unlikely to be able to explain this and other characteristics of these cells. It is noteworthy that the ratio changes from 2 to 1 when a rotating stimulus is used and its velocity increases from 2°/s to 20°/s, but the significance of these observations is still a riddle, though probably related to a connection between contrast sensitivity and exposure time.

The receptive field in retina and cortex

Cartesians (i.e. followers of the French philosopher Réné Descartes who believed the soul to be located in the brain) will learn with regret that the cerebral residence of perception has not been pinpointed. But area 17 contains cells which recognize short linear elements with specific orientations. In order to incorporate this functional aspect of a morphological entity, we have to look at the concept of the receptive field. Suppose that the eye of an experimental animal faces a screen. Stimuli can be projected thereon, and their shape and velocity is variable. These stimuli are, of course, imaged on the retina of the eye in question: if binocular stimulation is studied then both retinae have to receive images, a matter easier to arrange in predator animals, such as cats, than in herbivores like rabbits. Suppose further that a micro-electrode is inserted into a ganglion cell: the knowledge that this is so is based on a combination of circumstances, e.g. the type of potential elicited by a stimulus, coupled with specific staining studies which lead to the potential being identified as a sort of cellular signature tune. If the cell responds to photic stimuli in general, then the screen is scanned with a small stimulus so that one can establish at which point in the visual field the cell is looking. If the eye is immobilized then the co-ordinates of this point can be related e.g. to the position of the blind spot in the visual field, that is to say one can identify the part of the photo-receptor layer which informs the ganglion cell under test. In practice it is found that, if the stimulus is somewhat displaced, the cell will still respond. This procedure can be repeated, and a locus can be determined which covers all the points in the visual field, capable of eliciting a response from one particular cell: this locus defines its receptive field.

The response may be due to the onset of the stimulus and/or to its cessation: this determines whether it is an on- or an off-response (Fig. 1.33). Many receptive fields of ganglion cells are approximately circular and may have an on-centre with an off-surround, or *vice versa*. Fields due to neighbouring cells can, of course, overlap. Note that, once the visual response has reached the bipolar layer, it does not take the form of a graded potential, but is saltatory, i.e. it occurs in discrete all-or-none spikes of constant amplitude. As in other nervous messages, intensity is expressed in terms of the number of spikes and/or the rate of their discharge.

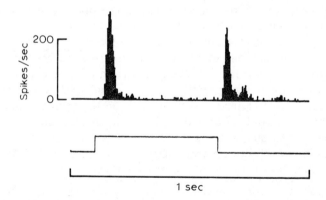

Fig. 1.33   On-off response of a pigeon ganglion cell to a spot flashed at the centre of the receptive field. Spike calibration of 200 spikes/sec correspond to 25.6 counts/bin. Bin-width 4 msec; 250 bins. (A bin is defined as the smallest possible receptacle of counted items, in this case: spikes.) Test spot and side spot 0.5° in diameter, and luminance 109 cd/sq m; background luminance 27 cd/sq m. The timing of the spot is indicated below. (1 cd/sq m is the luminance of a source emitting a luminous flux of 1 lumen per unit solid angle per square metre. 1 lumen is the luminance flux of power 0.00146 w at a wavelength of 555 nm.) (After Holden, 1977.)

However, another feature of cell discharges relates to their duration in comparison to that of the stimulus. Enroth-Cugell and Robson (1966) made a detailed study of optical factors of the eye of the cat, and accompanied this by an examination of ganglion discharges which they were able to subdivide into two broad classes. Depending on whether spatial summation within the receptive field was linear or not, they identified them as X or Y cells, later associated with moderate and fast conduction velocities. Not quite the same division applies to the rabbit. Its ganglion cells can be subdivided into X and Y cells, typified by sustained and transient discharges respectively (Fig. 1.34). About one quarter of the cells are of the on/off type. The rate of discharge leads the above and other authors to identify in both X and Y groups some 'sluggish' units. Another 25 per cent are direction sensitive, with the remainder orientation-selective, sensitive to local edges, large fields, and to featureless stimuli. It will be interesting to establish whether the complicated responses of cat retinal ganglion cells to intermittent stimuli can be correlated with the above classes of cell (Foerster *et al.*, 1977a, b). Similar cells have been identified in the retina of the macaque monkey, where they have significant chromatic properties. The majority exhibit a centre-surround organization. Chromatically, they may belong typically to the 'opponent-colour' system: for example, the centre may respond preferentially to red light and the surround to a complementary green. Or similar types of cone may be linked to different degrees with both the centre and the surround. Fig. 1.35 shows profiles of the sensitivity distribution of a pure centre/pure surround cell: the surround elements contributing to discontinuities when an additional test-spot was added to the pattern, as shown, were confined to the centre of the receptive field: note the Y-characteristics (de Monasterio, 1978a, b).

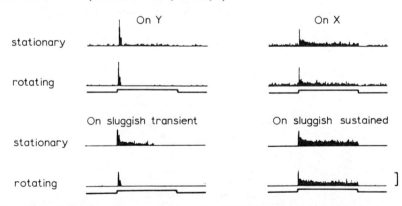

Fig. 1.34a Inhibition of the response of a rabbit ganglion cell to a central spot by rotation of a radial grating. The spot was on while the trace beneath the histogram was shifted upward. The grating was on continuously and either stationary during the entire histogram or rotating during the entire programme. The spot size was rather smaller than the centre of the receptive field. The grating was masked from an area rather larger than the centre of the receptive field: 24 sectors to the grating. There is a large effect of rotation upon the sluggish transient cell and some effect upon the Y cell: the small sustained component was eliminated by rotation of the grating and the transient slightly reduced. Y and sluggish transient cells: the calibration scale is 250 spikes/sec and the light was on 2 sec. X and sluggish sustained cells: the calibration scale is 125 spikes/sec and the light was on 4 sec. (From Caldwell and Daw, 1978. © The Physiological Society.)

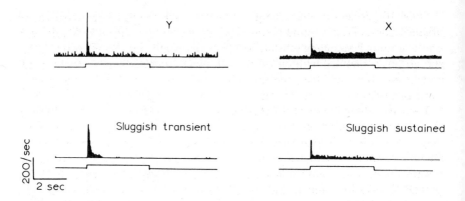

Fig. 1.34b   Response of a rabbit ganglion cell to a stationary white spot in the centre of the receptive field. Peri-stimulus time histograms. The initial section of each record is prestimulus. The spot was on while the trace beneath the histograms was shifted upward. The last part of the record is post-stimulus. All cells were on-centre. Both the Y cell and the sluggish transient cell had very transient responses, but the Y cell had a higher maximum frequency of firing and more spontaneous activity than the sluggish cell. The X cell had a higher and more regular spontaneous activity than either the Y cell or the sluggish sustained cell. (From Caldwell and Daw, 1978. © The Physiological Society.)

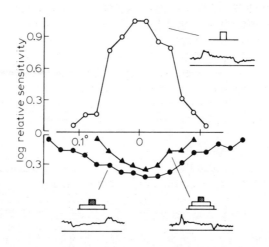

Fig. 1.35   Profiles of the spatial distribution of pure centre (open circles), pure surround (solid circles), and of mixed responses (solid triangles) of a type IV cell. Centre profile obtained with a 540 nm spot of 0.01° (nominal) on a white background of 150 td. Surround profile of pure responses obtained with a 600-nm spot of 0.03° on a 500 nm background $(4.2 \times 10^{10}$ quanta. s^{-1}. $deg^{-2})$. Mixed-response profile based on the threshold for a transient discontinuity in cell firing elicited by the concurrent flashing of a 540 nm spot of 20° and a 620 nm spot of 0.03° in the presence of a 500 nm background of 8.2×10^{7} quanta. s^{-1}. deg^{-2}. Pulse density tracings show representative averaged responses used to generate profiles. (From De Monasterio, 1978b. © The American Physiological Society, Bethesda.)

Some 10 per cent of macaque ganglion cells lack the usual centre-surround organizations, and are found predominantly outside the central area, although one group, not responding to white light, was frequently noted in the fovea. Other sub-groups responded with on/off to both small and large stimuli exciting red- and green-, but not blue-, sensitive cones. Others, again, responded only to moving targets imaged perifoveally (de Monasterio, 1978c).

There is nothing special about the concept of the receptive field outlined above. It is worth noting in passing that, e.g. in lower animals such as frogs, ganglion cells may be specialized in that they may have lower thresholds for some types of stimulus configuration than for others. In higher animals, specialization is pushed toward the nervous centre (but see above). This is a special example of a fairly general observation, namely that so-called higher species are characterized by a more highly integrated nervous system (and, therefore, behaviour), an arrangement which is, at one and the same time, more plastic, more adaptable, and less stereotyped. It is consequently more amenable to evolutionary benefits, and helps to explain why the higher species have become higher.

Inside the cortex

Since the receptive field is defined in the (external) visual field, it is clearly of interest to determine what shapes and characteristics it assumes when micro-electrodes are inserted not just into retinal ganglion cells but any other cell of the visual path, including the visual cortex. It cannot be taken for granted that it is immutable. Indeed, if the filter concept outlined on pp. 8–10 for the retina has general validity, then the complexity of the visual system would be quite pointless: if the information at cortical level had the same band-width and noise components as at the retinal stage then a lot of nervous and chemical energy would appear to fulfil no conceivable objective. However, some of the most imaginative experimentation in the field of vision, largely associated with the names of Hubel and Wiesel, shows that we need have no fear on this account. Their work is summarized in the Ferrier lecture (1977), and a cruel editor of the Royal Society stresses that, though it was delivered in 1972, the manuscript was not received till four years later.

In general, the neurones of the visual cortex are made up of columns with axes perpendicular to the cortical surface. Both columns and rows (i.e. the tangential distribution) exhibit a systematic variation as regards binocular representation, orientational sensitivity and so on. It does not seem that this columnar arrangement is specific to the visual cortex: it is also met e.g. in the central representation of the vibrissae of the mouse. It is too early to say whether it is developed whenever a two-dimensional surface used for the detection of a variety of stimulus modes is represented on the cortex or on one of its homologues.

Hubel and Wiesel (1962) discovered cells in the cat cortex which responded specifically to short slits oriented in a given direction (± 10–$20°$) and moving in one sense without responding when the sense was reversed (Fig. 1.36). These orientation detectors can, in combination, serve as pattern and movement detectors, and, as such, constitute a developmental advance over retinal ganglion cells and the cells of the lateral geniculate body, the receptive fields of which are approximately radially symmetrical in shape and function. In both the feline and

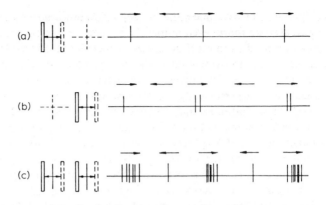

Fig. 1.36   Movement of a 1/4° × 2° slit back and forth horizontally across the receptive field of a binocularly influenced cell. a, left eye; b, right eye; c, both eyes. The cell clearly preferred left-to-right movement (note that B has a shorter latent period than does A), but when both eyes were stimulated together it responded also to the reverse direction. Field diameter, 2° situated 5° from the area centralis. Time, 1 sec. (From Hubel and Wiesel, 1962. © The Physiological Society.)

the primate cortex all orientational cells appear with approximately equal frequencies, but not all the cells are equally sensitive to particular orientations. Classifying cells in an ascending order of response diversity, Hubel and Wiesel distinguished in the cortex (a) circularly symmetric, (b) simple, (c) complex, and (d) hypercomplex units. These form probably a hierarchy, (a) receiving their input from the lateral geniculate nucleus. (b) shows a preference for position: if it changes even in the absence of an orientational modification, the response can alter. (c) behaves conversely more sensitively to the orientation than to the position of a line segment within the receptive field (RF) and is insensitive to diffuse light, i.e. radiation covering the whole of RF. (d) is similar to (c) except that an extension of the longest line producing a response abolishes its response. The specificity e.g. of orientation-sensitive neurones is reduced by the iontophoretic injection of bicuculline. This counteracts inhibition, e.g. that exerted by GABA (γ-aminobutyric acid), a putative neurotransmitter widely present in the central nervous system and, notably, also in the visual system. Facilitation, or the reduction of inhibition, generally leads to an impairment of nervous control, witness the effect of alcohol e.g. on the electro-retinogram and not only on the electro-retinogram.

As regards the ocular origin of the input, (a) and (b) are exclusively monocular, but binocular stimulation can be detected in about half of the (c) and (d) cells. It is noteworthy that, in binocular responses, the responses from either eye match each other virtually in all respects, so providing a physiological basis for the perceptual existence of the monocular cyclopean eye (in man). But this match is generally only qualitative in nature. Quantitatively there may be differences which find expression in the concept of ocular dominance, and, since about half of the cells are monocular, a one-sided input forms an extreme of this quantitative variation, the general pattern being genetically determined i.e. independent of visual experience. It is likely that the balance of the input from the two eyes is controlled at least in part by intra-cortical inhibition.

The cortex, in all 2 mm thick, is sub-divided morphologically into six layers (I–VI), some of which are further sub-divided (Fig. 1.37). Its thickness remains uniform even though the area devoted to foveal representation is relatively far greater than is true of the retinal periphery. The ratio of mm cortex/degree visual field is referred to as magnification F. The term is less unfortunate than it might seem as a result of its mixture of units because there is a simple relation between the extent of the visual field and its imaged extent on the retina if we exclude the retinal annulus near the ora serrata. Here the focal distance clearly can no longer be considered and the simple proportionality valid for the central area no longer obtains.

If a micro-electrode penetrates the cortex perpendicularly to its surface, it contacts cells with RF's which all overlap. Cells with the smallest fields are encountered in layer IVc, those with the largest RF's in layer V. Now if the electrode traverses the grey matter tangentially, a tip displacement of 1–2 mm leads it into a neighbouring, different cell aggregate: it follows from the previous paragraph that such a constant displacement corresponds to very different retinal areas depending on whether the cortical region probed is projected on to by the retinal centre or periphery.

An examination of the above-mentioned layers shows that the radially symmetric cells (a) are found mainly in layer IVc which contains those afferent terminals of the optic radiations not reaching layers I, IVb and VI. Simple cells (b) diminish in the neighbouring layer IVb and perhaps in VI, but complex and hypercomplex cells, (c) and (d), were observed in layers II, III, V, and VI. Furthermore, the cells in layer IVc are almost wholly monocular in input: this still holds partly for layer IVb, whereas layer II, III, V and VI contain more than 50 per cent binocular ones.

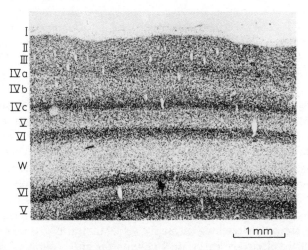

Fig. 1.37 Cross-section through the monkey striate cortex showing conventional layering designations. W, white matter. Deeper layers (VI, V) of the buried fold of cortex are shown in the lower part of the figure. Cresyl violet stain. (From Hubel and Wiesel, 1977. © 1977 The Royal Society, London.)

Ocular dominance varies systematically. A 'vertical' penetration shows that all the receptive fields exhibit approximately the same type of ocular dominance. For example, if cells in II are stimulated strongly by the right eye, but also (weakly) by the left one, this pattern will recur throughout the column, except, of course, that IV cells will be stimulated only by the right eye. This arrangement, columnar for ocular preference, has been found, so far, only in species with partial decussation of the optic nerves, and may be a correlate of frontal vision. Further, there is one systematizing the orientational sensitivity of the cortical cells. These are the cells the response of which is illustrated in Fig. 1.38. In the rabbit, direction selective detectors were discovered at the retinal level: their directions of maximal response clustered in three groups approximately at angles of 120° to one another, an arrangement of advantage to an animal that wishes to orientate *itself*.

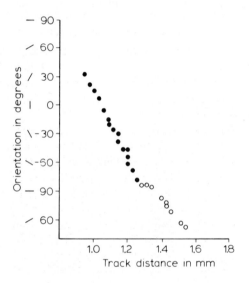

Fig. 1.38   Example of orientation in degrees plotted against electrode track distance in millimetres, ●, cells dominated by right eye; ○, left eye. (From Hubel and Wiesel, 1977. © 1977 The Royal Society, London.)

But in visually more developed species, such as primates, specialization has moved centripetally (cf. p. 42), and the orientation sensitivity resides in cortical neurones of types (c) and (d), as we noted on p. 45. Just as is true of dominance columns, micro-electrodes penetrating the cortex perpendicularly to its surface encounter cells with parallel axes of preferred direction. But whereas neighbouring dominance columns vary with their preferences in a 'streaky' manner, the orientational signature of a column changes systematically as is revealed in penetrations of the cortex done obliquely (Fig. 1.38). Note that the orientational network presumably stretching across the visual cortex reveals no discontinuity when the micro-electrode leaves an R-column for an L-column. The preferred axes turn through 180° every mm along the cortex, probably in steps of 10° (cf. p. 45). The ocular dominance streaks are approximately parallel and roughly 0.4 mm in width.

This remarkable result was obtained with four independent techniques:

(i) axons that have degenerated can be selectively stained, a method applicable following lesions in either of the lateral geniculate bodies;

(ii) nearly tangential electrode penetrations were combined with a special silver stain technique, while lesions were being made every time the electrode tip crossed from one preference column into another;

(iii) by the injection of radio-active label into the monkey's vitreous humour, which was carried as far as layer IVc (Fig. 1.39);

(iv) in animals injected intravenously with radio-active glucose, silver grains accumulate in previously active cells so that the closure or removal of one eye reveals in area 17 patterns of dominance columns which, in distinction from (iii), are exposed across all six layers.

It would seem, then, that the primate cortex is based on ocular dominance columns of alternating inputs and, within each of these, there are narrow slabs of like orientational preference, changing slab by slab by about 10°. Hubel and Wiesel have not, so far, given details of the organisation of detectors of other attributes of the retinal image such as colour or velocity. As regards the latter, one

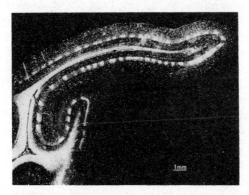

Fig. 1.39 A dark-field autoradiograph of striate cortex in an adult macaque in which the ipsilateral eye had been injected with tritiated proline-fucose 2 weeks before. The labelled areas appear white. The section passes for the most part in a plane perpendicular to the surface. The photograph shows part of the exposed surface of the striate cortex and the buried part immediately beneath; some of the buried part has fallen away during sectioning. In all, some 56 columns can be counted in layer IVc. (From Hubel and Wiesel, 1977. © 1977 The Royal Society, London.)

would expect very different systems in animals with frontal and lateral eyes respectively: a running rabbit has the world gliding past it all in the same direction, and this may enable it to gauge velocity. But a cat pouncing on a mouse may have to gauge (visual) velocity from the rate of enlargement of the retinal image, and unlike the rabbit, cannot rely on the mutual reinforcement of the rate of stimulation of orientation detectors with preferred axes pointing in similar directions. We have already observed that, in the cat and rabbit, this particular act of discrimination is carried out by special ganglion cells (p. 43). Recent studies suggest that man responds to velocity intrinsically, i.e. not by assessing the time that elapses when an object traverses two retinal loci that are a known (?) distance apart. With the existence of velocity detectors having been demonstrated the human intrinsic method needs contrast detection, but this clearly presents no problem.

In the cat, both cortical and geniculate neurones are distinguished from retinal ganglion cells in that their spatial frequency spectrum (cf. p. 15) barely varies with the luminance level of the stimulus over a range of four orders of magnitude. This would be expected if there is a direct input from the geniculate to cortical neurones. Complex cells (p. 46) are more sensitive to contrast at low luminance levels than is true of simple cells, but even at levels as low as 5×10^{-4} cd/sqm there is a specific depression at low spatial frequencies. In man, this low frequency depression is observed when the exposure time t is long (1 s), but vanishes when t $\sim$ 10 ms. The spatial frequency spectrum of complex cells also tends to be broader than that of simple cells (Fig. 1.40) the broadening being present on the high frequency side. Simple cells respond $4/\pi$ times more to low-frequency square gratings than to sinusoidal ones of the same frequency, presumably owing to the presence of the third harmonic revealed by Fourier analysis. If this component is subtracted, the resultant response is zero even though the stimulus contains discontinuities at the edges. These have high-frequency components to which simple cells are not sensitive, as has just been noted. Analogous observations made on the visibility of similar gratings show that the human visual system can respond in a like manner, and this observation is used to support the notion that it is served by channels selectively tuned to bands of spatial frequencies. Neurophysiologists are undecided to what extent this, and other parts of the visual process, are organized on serially hierarchic or parallel lines respectively.

In monkeys, simple cortical cells respond to each edge of moving square-wave gratings of low spatial frequency, and to pairs of edges when the frequency is high. But complex cells respond more diffusely. Tests with sine-wave gratings showed that, in both types of cell, the spatial frequency of maximum sensitivity $v$max decreases when areas remote from the fovea are sampled: whereas in the centre $v$max $\approx$ 4c/° or more, at a distance of 20° it is reduced to 1 c/°. v max showed a low but negative correlation with the size of the receptive field; however, in the case of cats, this correlation is extremely high for all kinds of cortical cell (Fig. 1.41) and, if this observation were generally valid, it would explain the above variation with eccentricity, observed in monkeys, as the size of the receptive field increases with the distance from the fovea.

Although the striate area was amongst the first to receive detailed attention – probably on account of its accessibility as much to probing electrodes as to traumatic stimuli – the focus of interest has understandably shifted to less peripheral areas. This is particularly true of the pre-striate visual cortex. It turns out that area 17 projects into no fewer than four areas within the precincts of Brodmann's areas 18 and 19: these are referred to as V2, V3, V4, and a striate-receptive area, located in the superior temporal sulcus (Fig. 1.42). The various projections are not quantitative replicas of e.g. the retinal projection on the striate area with changed magnification factors F – where F (cf. p. 47) is the length along cortical surface per degree of visual (retinal) field – but represent the results of gating operations. They consequently subserve specialized functional modalities (see also Fig. 1.43a, b). Thus, a binocular disparity response is characteristic of cells in V2, specific chromatic stimuli are recorded from V4, and motion-sensitive cells

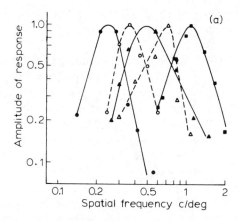

Fig. 1.40a Response of simple cat cortical cells to a sinusoidal grating, as a function of spatial frequency. The ordinates represent the amplitude of the averaged responses to the passage of a single period of the grating (bright + dark bar) over the cell receptive field. The maximal amplitude of response of each cell has been taken as 1. Average luminance of the grating 2 cd/m², contrast 20 per cent. The grating velocity was constant, of the order of 1–2°/sec. and chosen to maximize the cell response. Filled circles: unit with an on-centre region of 1.2° width, flanked by two off-regions. Total width of the receptive field 5°. Open circles: unit with a receptive field of the same type as the previous one, but with very weak off flanks. On centre region of 1° width. Filled triangles: unit with a bipartite receptive field consisting of an on-region of 1.3° flanked by one off-region of 0.7° width. Open triangles: unit with a bipartite receptive field of total width 0.9°. Filled squares: unit with a bipartite receptive field of total width 0.6°. (After Maffei and Fiorentini, 1973.)

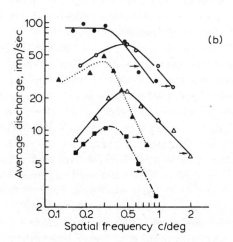

Fig. 1.40b Ditto for complex cells. The ordinates represent the average discharge of the cell evaluated over 1 min period while the grating was moving at constant velocity over the cell receptive field. The velocity was such as to maximize the cell discharge and was of the order of several °/sec. Other experimental conditions as for Fig. 1.40a. Width of the receptive field: 6° (filled circles), 5° (open circles), 3° (filled triangles), 1.5° (open triangles), 3° (filled squares). The arrows indicate the average discharge of the cell in the absence of the stimulus. Note the difference in band-width as between simple and complex cells (After Maffei and Fiorentini, 1973.)

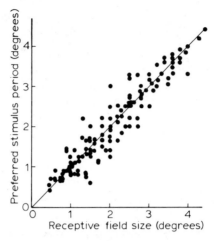

Fig. 1.41 Correlation between receptive field size and preferred spatial period for 120 cat cortical neurons (simple, complex and hypercomplex) in area 17. The receptive field was mapped for simple and hypercomplex neurons: it included both excitatory and inhibitory regions. The receptive field size (abscissa) was measured in the direction perpendicular to the preferred orientation of the cell. The correlation coefficient for this population of cells is 0.94 and the computed regression line has a slope of 0.97. (After Maffei and Fiorentini, 1977.)

dominate in the striate-receptive area of the superior temporal sulcus. At the same time, one has to appreciate the topographic problem of mapping a highly convoluted area of cortex: the sulcus is curved both longitudinally and, with much higher curvatures, laterally: a two-dimensional representation is going to be useful in that it reproduces *relations* between points without, of course, giving an unambiguous indication of inter-point distances.

When interhemispheric connections passing through the corpus callosum are sectioned, degenerate fibres are later found to terminate along the border between striate and prestriate areas (VI/V2) and in the lunate, the annectant and the parieto-occipital sulci. The V1/V2 complex has maps in register over the region where the two areas are closely apposed; in fact, a small lesion in VI leads to degeneration in V2, so confirming their connection. But the receptive field-size is larger in V2: the F-value is increased. The contralateral visual field is represented in a newly-discovered area V3A, and in V4, and each area contains multiple representations of several parts of the visual field. In the cat, the spatial frequency responses of cells in area 18 shows systematic differences from those in area 17 even though the layering parallel to the cortical surface is approximately maintained. Thus the maximum of the contrast sensitivity curve is at a lower frequency in area 18, as is true of the resolving power. As in area 17, cells located in the same (tangential) layer have the same maximum frequency and bandwidth, while the orientation varies in adjacent columns as shown in Fig. 1.38. The differences between the response characteristics of the two areas may result in part from the fact that X-cells feed information predominantly into area 17, whereas Y-cells do so for area 18. Almost all the cells in the above areas could be driven binocularly from either eye: whether this is significant from the point of

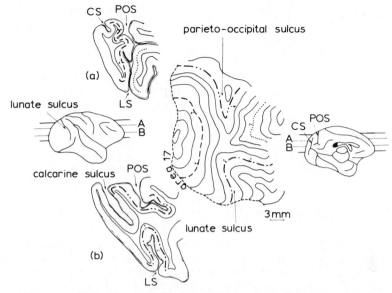

Fig. 1.42   A method of constructing a two-dimensional 'unfolded' cortical map of the prestriate cortex. Drawings of representative sections at two horizontal levels are shown in the upper and lower left corners. In the more dorsal section (a, upper left) the contour followed by layer IV was divided into separate posterior (— — —) and anterior (. . . . . .) sections. The shape of each contour was then changed slightly in order to fit into the composite cortical map (centre). In the more ventral section (b, lower left) layer IV contours are divided into separate lateral (—, —, —) and medial (— —·· — —··) sections. The figure shows the re-construction of the right prestriate cortex. W to Z etc. are location marks. Sections (a), (b) = planes A, B. (After Van Essen and Zeki, 1978.)

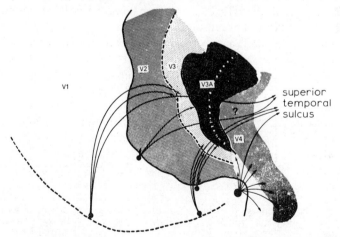

Fig. 1.43a   Synthetic diagram of the projections of the striate cortex, based on information obtained in a number of studies. Interrupted lines indicate the representation of the horizontal meridian, continuous lines that of the vertical meridian. The gap between the superior temporal sulcus (STS) and the other prestriate areas depicted here refers to the surface of the prelunate gyrus an the lateral part of the posterior bank of the STS. Only the projections of the part of the striate cortex representing lower visual fields are shown. (After Zeki, 1978a.)

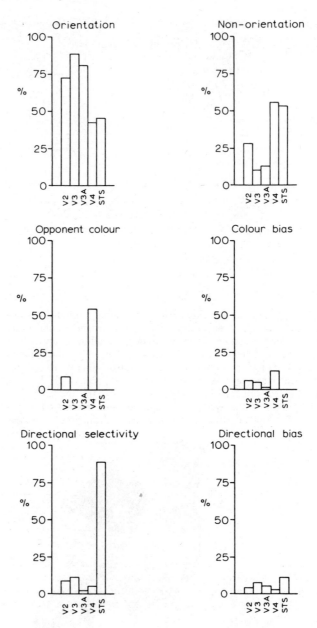

Fig. 1.43b The percentage distribution of orientation selective, colour selective, and directionally sensitive cells in five prestriate areas. (From Zeki, 1978c. © The Physiological Society.)

view of binocular vision can only be determined when a part of the non-overlapping field of the eye is used as a control. The problem of stereopsis (or binocular depth perception) can only be tackled in terms of binocular cells detecting retinal disparity (p. 159).

The foveal projections of the striate cortex of the rhesus monkey are distinguished from extra-foveal ones in an important qualitative respect: a point 3° below the fixation area projects to the lunate sulcus (V2 and V3) and to the movement areas of the posterior bank of the superior temporal sulcus. A basically similar pattern emerges when a lesion is made from the striate projection of a point 2° above the fixation area. This is also true for the foveal projection, but, in addition, the field of degenerate fibres spreads over the anterior bank of the lunate sulcus, right up to the prelunate gyrus, which is occupied by V4 (Zeki, 1978a). Fig. 1.43 indicates some of the multiple projections from the striate to other areas: in view of the functional separation of these areas (cf. p. 52), we can conclude that this is mediated by a physical gating process.

A remarkable, and so far unexplained, observation relates to the double representation of visual fields in areas V3 and V3A of the rhesus cortex (Zeki, 1978b) with cells that are all binocularly driven, unspecialized as regards colour, and all orientation sensitive. It represents, however, a clear example of pathways usable in parallel as distinct from serial information processing, and stresses that a great deal has yet to be learnt from the discharge sequences occurring as far peripherally as the optic nerve. That parallel processing may involve a division of labour transpires also from studies of the frequency distribution of modalities (Zeki, 1978c). Fig. 1.43 shows that chromatic responses reveal almost perfect specialization in area V4 even though V2 represents the central 5° of the visual fields examined in that study. The dominance of directional selectivity in the superior temporal sulcus may make this area a centre concerned with the detection of motion: an electrode implanted in this region could test this view e.g. in experiments in which eye movements are examined as a result of the movement of targets in the visual field.

And so it will continue. Not *ad infinitum*, of course, for not even the immense number of brain cells makes it likely that area will project onto area. In the first place, the mere existence of reflexes shows that there are paths leading to efferent systems, like the superior colliculi, or the oculo-motor nuclei. Some of them remain to be traced in detail. Secondly, we ought to consider the brain from a more outward-looking point of view. As noted above, neurophysiologists measure magnification factors, i.e. the ratios of a distance along a more central part of the brain to one along a more peripheral part, it being remembered that, embryologically speaking, the retina is an outcrop of the developing brain. Now if one adopts a cerebrocentric as distinct from a retinocentric point of view, then the mode of thinking has to be changed: we start with a wealth of cells at the centre, and a handful of them are sent out as ambassadors beyond the skull to report on what is going on outside. Although the change from magnification factors to minification or reduction factors involves quantitatively only reciprocals, it raises interesting questions for comparative morphology. For example with area V4 acting as a chromatic relay centre, one will want to know whether all species with colour vision have a homologous area, whether V4 exists in higher animals with relatively little or no colour vision, whether it is 'set aside' when cones develop with different pigments in them, whether it exists in colour-defective individuals etc. It is not inevitable that the optical differentiation of a stimulus leads to the need for its neural counterpart: the argument is merely the result of one particular view of information processing, namely the serial variety. Parallel processing may develop along centrifugal lines, which may be illustrated by the following example.

Suppose there is a brain that has learnt to accumulate disconnected place names. We might say, by analogy with some of the cells mentioned above, that it has an area A1 containing 'ordinate' cells, one of them recording that London stands for 52°N 0°E. If it has no other type of cell, it will not understand why Paris differs from London. Hence a Hamlet would ruminate along the lines of: 'To—or not to—'. But then, since curiosity seems to be a prime mover during one phase of cerebral development, some cortical cells might propel neural pseudopodia (or messengers) to the retina. The cortical cells in area A2 would learn to put two and two together and the idea of relation would develop. Hamlet would learn to ruminate 'To be or not to be', and the 'relational' cells would combine with the parallel informational content of the ordinate cells to allow a projection area A3 of the two to conclude that London *is* north of Paris. A micro-electrode probing A1 would record a discharge whenever the retina was presented with a place name. A2 would respond to movement. Then A3, which clearly has at least one attribute of mind, would respond to either of the two stimuli. But the discharge pattern would not allow us to draw any other conclusion. We have to ask ourselves whether our quest is to discover how we see, or how we know that we *are* seeing, or – most likely – how we know that *we* are seeing. The line between the realization of perception and self-consciousness may be thin. It is not established that existing methods, let alone electrophysiology, can determine where it is.

But these pages are supposed to deal with physiology, not philosophy. And the visual system is one worthy of our attention on account of its intrinisic interest even if, defying Descartes, it may not allow us to catch a glimpse of our soul.

Questions

1 Someone has lost one of his crystalline lenses as a result of an accident. The eye in question has fortunately not suffered in any other way. He measures his spectral sensitivity curve at an extremely low luminance level with each eye in turn. What information can you obtain from the two sets of data?

2 How can studies of the ERP provide information on eye disease? In the diagnosis of what diseases is it likely to be particularly informative, and how would you set about obtaining and interpreting the information?

3 You have impaled a cell in area 17 and are obtaining photic responses. How would you study what effect alcohol has on function when it is applied to (a) the retina, (b) the lateral geniculate body, (c) the cortex? Would you expect any difference? If so, why?

4 Explain what is meant by receptive field. How does it fit into the concept of the eye being a filtering system for information?

2 Light as a Governor

Whenever we think about eyes we see them as organs of vision. They signal danger at a distance, pressures in proximity, food before us; it is by their aid that we move our limbs, control our bodily posture, steer our cars and aircraft; in short, they process the available photic information, and transmit a studied selection to the brain.

Yet we have to face the question of whether this is the sum total of their function – both in man and animals, or whether a fraction of the visual load may not perhaps be used to control bodily functions which are involuntary without being part of the physiologist's concept of autonomy. The cycles of day and night, and of working and sleeping, are so much part of our nature as to make us forget how they rule the conduct of our affairs. And while light quanta cannot be aware of whether they are the harbingers of wars or whether they act perhaps like time-switches, it is an objective of sound research to obtain an answer to this intriguing problem.

Some physiological clocks have been known for a long time. As a rule we sleep when it is dark, and wake in the light. Our body temperature varies from a minimum at about 03.00 hours to a maximum at 16.00 hours, a circumstance long known to doctors watching patients in a fever. Venous pressure is minimal at about 08.00 hours and rises to a maximum at 22.00 hours. On the other hand, intraocular pressure drops from a high level at about 09.00 hours to a low in the afternoon with a subsidiary peak at about noontime. Pupil dilation which reduces outflow facility clearly distorts the 'normal' cycle at night (Fig. 2.1). What is the

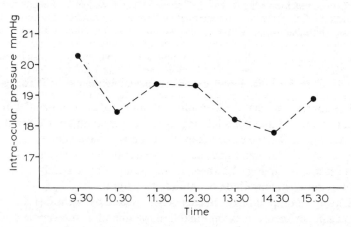

Fig. 2.1 The variation in intra-ocular pressure over a period of six hours. (From Gloster, 1966. © Churchill Livingstone, Edinburgh.)

origin of these and other rhythms to be mentioned below? Is there a prime-mover, some Aristotelian lever that turns our individual universes once every twenty-four hours? Is there some innate primeval pendulum that swings through the body and rings bells at various times in various places? What if – dreaded possibility – there is mutual interaction between some glandular stimulation in one tissue and inhibition in another? Just as no man is an island so no tissue can exist for long in isolation. The study of circadian rhythms (*circa* = approximately, *dies* = day) is a nightmare because the scientist's ideal, namely the isolation of the complex under test, almost always destructively interferes with the system as a whole.

The physiological stimulus

These are some of the reasons why appeal to rather obvious statistics is of no avail. On the face of it, there is a drastic difference between the temporal and spatial distribution of light quanta forming images and so carrying 'bits' of information on the one hand, and the blanket of light governing ambient illumination on the other. They are, of course, easy enough to distinguish from each other especially on an objective basis. After all, the mammalian cortex contains specialized cells (p. 172) which are particularly sensitive to patterned illumination, but barely sensitive to diffuse light, much as some lower vertebrates, such as the frog, have retinae with feature-sensitive ganglion cells (p. 36) but also possess the specialized, or rudimentary, third eye (stirnorgan) which responds to background light.

However, whereas such systems can be effectively singled out and analysed, a causal chain with environmental influences is hard to establish with confidence. There are surprisingly few biologists devoting their energy to the study of circadian rhythms who have appreciated the difficulty presented by the possibility of diurnal variations not in the intensity of external stimuli but in systemic sensitivity. One of those few is F. A. Brown (1959) who put forward the interesting notion of 'auto-phasing' in the following way:

> The organism reaching a 'light-sensitive' phase in its daily cycle, and encountering the illumination of a constantly illuminated environment, would be given a shifting stimulus whose strength, within limits, would be a function of the level of the illumination. Though physically the light is held constant, in stimulative effectiveness for the organism it is rhythmic as a consequence of rhythms in the organism's own responsiveness . . . This may depend upon the character of the daily rhythm of sensitivity of the particular species or individual, and hence may be in part genetic.

It will be appreciated that the 'constantly illuminated environment' is artificial in most latitudes, and that it is a laboratory device for eliminating diurnal photic intensity variations. By the same token, Brown might have added that constant darkness could act in an analogous manner on a system which responds actively to a zero stimulus: in Fig. 2.2 there is an example of a steady background discharge, reduced in amplitude or inhibited by light.

Brown's important point has been severely criticized by Aschoff (1963), but the original argument seems unexceptionable if we abandon the simple notion of stimulus. This is generally a quantity of radiation, or a number of quanta, but it

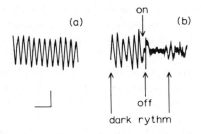

Fig. 2.2 Dark oscillations. Cat, presphenoidal exposure of tract. (a) steady oscillations at about 3/s after some 10 s in the dark; (b) overhead lights switched on and off momentarily ('off' indicated by large artifact) disrupting rhythm. Amplitude calibration, 200 μV: time, 1 s. (From Doty and Kimura, 1963. © The Physiological Society.)

gives limited information if it is unrelated to the organism's response to it. A large dose of radio-waves has no visual effect because the retina does not absorb them (p. 26). It is pointless to think here in terms of sub-threshold stimuli because it is unlikely that a monochromatic source radiating in the giga-Hz range with such an intensity as to stimulate the eye is going to be realized. Brown's argument becomes self-evident if stimuli are expressed not only in the appropriate physical units but also as multiples (or sub-multiples) of the relevant threshold. For example to be told that the human eye can detect three, two, or even one quantum tells us a lot about the sensitivity of our photo-receptors. In some ways, it is even more informative that the visual range is 10^{12} threshold units, i.e. that the greatest stimulus capable of evoking a differential visual sensation is a million million times greater than that able to evoke the least sensation of all. We arrive therefore at the concept of the effective stimulus I(eff) which is biophysically more useful than the single radiometric value I(r):

$$I(eff) = I(r)/I(th) \qquad \textbf{2.1}$$

where I(th) is the absolute threshold. It is not essential, of course, to use the absolute threshold as a standard, as long as some threshold value is employed. In fact, the use of intensity units involves a number of assumptions which cannot always be substantiated. It is, therefore, more appropriate to express stimuli in terms not of radiation flux (i.e. intensity) but in those of the quantity of radiation. This can then be assimilated to quanta of action (see p. 28).

The sensitivity of an organism is defined as the reciprocal of the threshold: this has the advantage that a high performance can be expressed with a high number rather than vice versa. If this substitution is made, then

$$I(eff) = I(r) \times S \qquad \textbf{2.2}$$

Suppose now that the amplitude of the stimulus I(r) varies with a frequency v where $v = 1/\tau$, τ being the period. Then

$$I(eff) = I'(r) \times (\cos 2\pi v t)^2 \times S \qquad \textbf{2.3}$$

where the primed value is the maximum of I(r) and t is the time. This is indistinguishable from

$$I(eff) = I'(r) \times S' \times (\cos 2\pi v t)^2 \qquad \textbf{2.4}$$

i.e. from a system responding with a periodically varying sensitivity to a constant stimulus. And this represents Brown's valid point in a formal manner.

The situation is complicated by yet another factor. This is best illustrated by a typical example of a circadian rhythm. It is possible to record the number of revolutions per hour caused on a wheel e.g. by two species of doormouse (*Peromyscus maniculatus* and *leucopus*) and the golden hamster (*Mesocricetus auratus*). Appropriate data obtained under conditions of equally long light and dark periods (LD = 12:12) are shown in Fig. 2.3. When the animals are released from this regime into darkness, the periodicity continues frequently at a changed 'free-running' level (Bünning, 1973). It is, therefore, not due to the direct effect of light although we shall see that even in a single neurone, light can establish a rhythm which the neurone 'remembers' for several days in the dark, albeit at a reduced amplitude. In 1974, Pittendrigh and Daan observed that the period varies systematically with age: it is shorter in older animals. Remember that, like most rodents, these species have rod-dominated retinae, and are active in the dark. Thus the observation that it is the older animals that are the first to emerge from their holes in the evening may be due to a factor unrelated to any endocrinological or metabolic influence whatsoever. A number of circumstances may conspire to

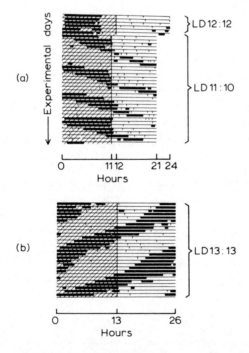

Fig. 2.3 Activity record of hamsters (*Mesocricetus auratus*, a nocturnal animal). (a) Synchronization by LD 12:12 hours (5 days). During the following 32 days (LD 11:10 hours) synchronization fails. The animal shows its individual free-running period of about 24.2 hours. During the days in which the animal's subjective night coincides with the light period, the activity is strongly suppressed by the light. Thus the animal has a few 'good' nights only in intervals of about one week. (b) LD 13:13 hours. Synchronization fails and the free-running periodicity becomes evident. Dark periods shaded. Light-intensity = 100 lux. (After Bünning, 1973.)

raise the visual threshold of older individuals so that the environment seems darker to them than to younger members of the species. As man, e.g., ages, the pupil becomes smaller and the lens absorbs more and more light (p. 133). This leads to a predictable rise in threshold (cf. Ch. 3). Yellowing of the lens occurs also in cats. It may be that wild animals do not live long enough for this to become significant, but pupillary miosis, if present, may manifest early in their lives. It is also possible that no miosis occurs in them. But the point to stress is that the full significance of Pittendrigh and Daan's observation of the senile variation in the rhythm of their rodents cannot be assessed in the absence of information on the visual thresholds of these animals. Eq. 2.2 tells us that, if S drops, I(eff) also drops: thus the older animals would experience darkness before the young ones do. They will also experience it longer and should return to their hideouts after their off-spring: however, the reverse is true. This may mean, however, nothing more than that the periods are similar in young and old, but that there is a phase change due, e.g., to a contribution of raised threshold and fatigue.

What is a stimulus?

It is impossible to overemphasize a kindred point frequently overlooked by chronobiologists: this relates to the precise definition of the stimulus. Specifying the latter in terms of illumination levels outside an animal's eyes is of limited value: what is physiologically more significant is the energy actually reaching, and being absorbed by, the retina. This requires a knowledge of the retinal illumination (Ch. 1). Hoffmann, to give an example, has compared the periods of activity of nocturnal animals like the mouse and the golden hamster as a function of the light intensity in the LL condition, i.e. in continuous light. The remarkable agreement between the two sets of data Fig. 2.4. obscures the fact that the optics of the two types of eye probably differ significantly, and that, in terms of threshold units (cf. p. 59) stimuli physically similar may, for different species, be physiologically different.

Again, while expatiating on stimulus control, Aschoff (1963) appears to overlook that, when a circadian rhythm is patent, [photic] synchronization operates by overkill. If it is of evolutionary significance it cannot be governed by a threshold stimulus, but it is just such a stimulus that is needed for the elucidation of a mechanism mediated by photo-receptors. This point is appreciated by Bünning (1973) who states clearly that 'higher intensities act faster' and that 'LD cycles are the most efficient synchronizers of circadian rhythms', and adds that 'in all cases the limits of entrainment will be reached earlier when working [sic] with rather low intensities'. But even this author stresses that natural light has to be used with circumspection on account of the variability of cloud cover etc! Practical advice points to the use of intensities between 1–10 lux (1 h before sunrise and $\frac{1}{2}$ h after sunset) as the best reference points for physiological measurement. Experts in vision would probably choose controllable artificial light.

None of these reservations can blind us to the significance of the study of circadian rhythms. Indeed, if their importance were not so widespread, one would not bother to express one's doubts. The role these rhythms play is not confined to academic interest in zoological curiosities. With Concorde flying approximately

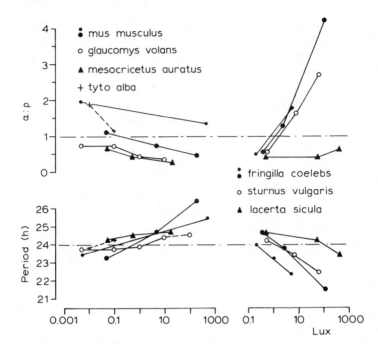

Fig. 2.4 Period and ratio of activity-time to rest-time $(\alpha:\rho)$ as a function of light-intensity in constant illumination. *Left*: four nocturnal species (mouse, flying squirrel, hamster, owl): *right*: three diurnal species (finch, starling, lizard). (After Hoffmann, 1965.)

at the speed with which the earth rotates, a day or night can assume bizarre proportions: jet-lag is due to an upset in our circadian rhythm. Again, people on night-shift who have to learn to transfer their activity peaks experience phase changes which – unlike the jet situation – involve continual priming.

Chronodons

These conditions raise the questions as to the extent, if any, to which some of our functions are programmed to perform with periodic variations, and, if so, whether they are subject to external governors or 'Zeitgebers', or chronodons as I propose to refer to them. The first point has familiar concomitants: if there are endogenous rhythms what are the relative contributions of nature and nurture respectively? Are there any social controls? Do the chronodons act as synchronizers to overcome the latitude or noise inherent in the individual rhythms when these are running freely?

Aschoff (1976) emphasizes in a useful and readable review that circadian rhythms assume a significance almost of one of the fundamental properties of biological matter. They are observed in unicellular marine algae as well as in a poly-cellular assembly such as man. They appear at enzymatic levels, in cells of all sorts, and can be revealed, as we shall note e.g. in connection with the retina, by radiographic methods. If present in individual cells, then evolutionary pressures would lead to one of several developments. Circadian rhythms would get lost in cell assemblies if they could not be synchronized, or else a master-clock might develop which, in turn, would be subject to some external control such as a chronodon might provide in terms of a light-dark or a hot-cold cycle. But even the attractive and simplifying concept of a master-clock is quickly disproved. If we postulate that the diurnal body-temperature change with its high in the afternoon and its low during the grey hours of the night is governed by our activity then we are in for a shock. In a free-running situation when day and night are illuminated, body temperature rises to a maximum two hours after waking and drops to its minimum when the individual begins his deep sleep. Even if some hormone or other acts like a master-clock, the coupling must be rather feeble if it is so easily undone.

Obviously, experiments on both sighted and blind people can provide some information as to how much control light may exert. A variety of physiological functions were monitored during midsummer voyages to the Arctic. In spite of significant changes, adaptation to 21 and 27 h days was uncommon, and was never complete even after six weeks. At latitudes when daylight became continuous, water excretion which normally reaches its maximum before noon and drops, possibly owing to training, to a minimum in the latter part of the night became desynchronized at first. However, the excretion of K^+ was frequently maintained. It may be that the small environmental fluctuations persisting in these regions even at the time of the summer solstice suffice to maintain this metabolic rhythm. After a fortnight, water excretion re-established a 24 h rhythm, the cause of which is unknown. Partially sighted subjects were shown to have a normal rhythm for water excretion, a matter for little surprise if we are looking for an explanation to the ambient illumination. However, the pattern for blind persons differed significantly. The amplitudes of the K^+, of Na^+ and Cl^- variations were reduced and there were notable phase shifts (Fig. 2.5). This raises the question whether the blind reveal the true circadian rhythms of these functions, unmodified by the chrono-control of the daily light-dark cycle. Aschoff (1976) reports on similar studies done on seven blind subjects, one of whom was congenitally so. This worker believes that social clues can provide powerful synchronization. A 24 h cycle in the rhythms of body temperature, urinary cortisol excretion (which is subject to renal rhythms, cf. p. 74) and other urinary solutes was maintained during the start of the experiment, even if within poorer limits than was true for sighted subjects. Aschoff attributes this initial correlation to social cues such as 'people came and went'. Later, when the subjects were isolated, the circadian rhythms extended to 25 h, in other words, persisted but with an extended period.

Time versus light

There seems little doubt that these studies agree on basic circadian rhythms differing in blind and sighted persons respectively. However, it is difficult to know what weight to ascribe to 'social' influence. It is not as though this factor can be quantified – one personal contact will have little less influence than will ten – and even the all-or-none effect, if any, has not been established beyond any shadow of doubt. In some ways, the young science of chronobiology is still

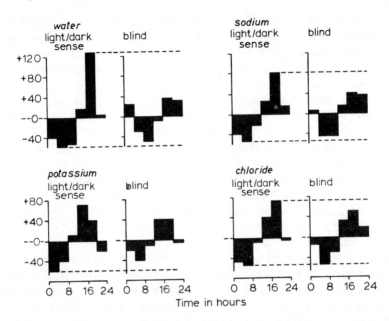

Fig. 2.5 Excretion of water, potassium, sodium and chloride by subjects with impaired vision. Comparison of the average values for five partially-sighted subjects (to the left of each plot) with those for five blind subjects. Excretory rates plotted as percentages about a mean: range of oscillation of excretory pattern indicated by horizontal interrupted lines. (From Lobban, 1965. © North Holland Publishing Co., Amsterdam.)

suffering from teething troubles. One has to return again and again to the considerable complications attending this study, and current metrological procedures testify to them. As the independent variable is physical time, one is obliged to face the question whether sampling ought to be done at random or at regular intervals, in view of the possibility that the latter may act as chronodons in their own right. But the determination of the dependent variable offers an even harder obstacle to surmount. The reasons are as follows.

Stimulus or response criteria?

In the observation of circadian rhythms one is generally concerned with responses of sorts. As we noted on p. 60, one determines e.g. the number of rotations per hour through which a rodent pedals a wheel at various times of a diurnal period. Although a free-run (LL) indicates the existence of a rhythm if there is a systematic periodic variation in the counts, the metrology of the experiments is unsatisfactory because they are uncalibrated. The fact of the matter is that, under natural conditions, it is not time that is the independent variable but the temporal variation of temperature or light intensity or humidity or some other environmental factor. Moreover, the biological noise in the contributory systems makes it impossible to determine the minimum conditions that will set up or desynchronize a rhythm. Although a voyage to the Arctic desynchronizes urinary excretion for a fortnight in sighted subjects, and the blind have different characteristics (p. 63), by how much does the normal light pattern have to change in the normal (a) to reveal minimal desynchronization and (b) to mimic the situation in the blind? One cannot take it for granted that the phase shifts in K^+, Na^+ and Cl^- excretion can be seen only in blind subjects unless an admittedly tiresome study at low-level illumination has first been carried out on normally sighted subjects. It may sound dogmatic to say that there is no obvious way round this problem; but the history of the physiology of vision is littered with casualties of reputations of those who thought that this could be done e.g. in connection with the quantification of responses in the visual system, not to mention visual sensations. There is no field involving behavioural responses wherein this hurdle has been surmounted unequivocally.

Experimental control

Promising control experiments have been attempted not only on animals but also on man. Yet unanimity as regards the interpretation of the data has been hard to come by probably because it is too difficult to obtain an adequate assessment of individual variations. For example Meddis (1968) studied how people adapt to a 48 h day, i.e. if, in the course of four weeks, they sleep on alternate nights. It turned out that, from the point of view of time spent on sleep, this arrangement was more economical: subjects slept during a quarter of the cycle as compared with one third (i.e. 8 h) in the control 24 h period. Body temperature variation was unaffected by the change in routine. Webb and Agnew (1975) varied the length of the sleep-wake cycle from 9 to 36 h, keeping the ratio constant at 1:2 over a period of four consecutive days. They found that the total loss of sleep was minimal at the 24 h value, suggesting, at variance with Meddis' result, that the 'normal' day is the most economic one. A heavy sleep deficit observed in men kept for 5–6 months in solitary underground confinement with self-controlled activity cycles and illumination is attributed to motivation and personality factors. Indeed, Wever says that desynchronization, and, therefore, differential effects due to various chronodons tend to occur in accentuated neuroses. Desynchronization is also observed in higher age groups, but as neuroses dominate in lower ones, more than one internally active synchronizing mechanism must clearly exist. If we are dealing with a difference due to the distinction in the definition of 'sleep', its relation to body temperature as explained by Meddis may need reconsidering. In fact, Wever has shown that circadian rhythms of man follow different courses depending on whether the (artificial) illumination in his photically isolated environment is or is not under the subject's control. There is, e.g., a phase shift in the spontaneous sleep-wake cycle under constant illumination (Fig. 2.6), in approximate synchrony with the minima and maxima of the body temperature, as indicated by the upright and inverted triangles respectively. An increase in ambient illumination on day 10 shortens the period as Aschoff first observed for diurnal animals. Again, if the illumination is kept on all the time, but reduced and increased on the days shown in Fig. 2.7, desynchronization between sleep/wake cycle and temperature rhythm occurs one week after the reduction, and remains unaffected by a subsequent rise in illumination. However, when subjects were allowed to switch off the room light on going to bed, desynchronization failed to

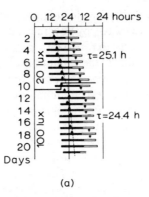

(a)

Fig. 2.6a Autonomous circadianism of a subject in constant illumination with an intensity variation. ▲ and ▼ represent maximum and minimum rectal temperatures respectively.

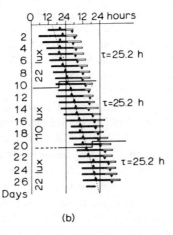

(b)

Fig. 2.6b Ditto, with two intensity variations. Symbols as in (a). Black bar: activity; white bar: resting period. (After Wever, 1969.)

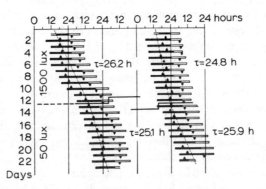

Fig. 2.7 Autonomic circadian periodicity of the same subject having the choice of time of illumination change; *left*: single subject; *right*: group test. Symbols as in Fig. 2.6. (After Wever, 1969.)

appear either when they were on their own or when à deux (Fig. 2.8). Wever showed that there is no significant correlation between level of illumination and duration of the circadian cycle. However, on balance, a negative correlation is observed in group tests, a positive one in isolation when switching off lights at 'bed-time' is permitted. When the illumination is maintained this pattern is only hinted at.

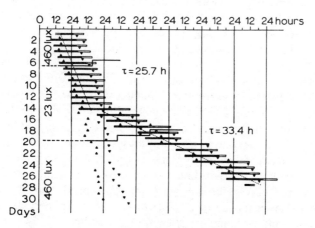

Fig. 2.8 Autonomous circadian periodicity of a subject in constant illumination with a two-fold change in illumination. Internal desynchronisation occurred on the 14th subjective day. Black triangles represent maximum and minimum rectal temperatures respectively (cf. Fig. 2.6a); white triangles merely repeat the positions of the black ones to correspond to the desynchronised time. (After Wever, 1969.)

The cross-currents set up by the sundry variables suffice to indicate that it will be difficult to obtain the sort of clear-cut answer looked for on p. 62. In particular, the effects of social cues are such as to complicate investigations into purely photic causes. When both physiological functions (rectal temperature, excretion of catecholamines, Na^+, and 17-hydroxycortico steroids) and psycho-motor characteristics (speed of tapping, time estimation, hand grip strength) were determined, there was no significant difference between three groups of two subjects living for four days in complete darkness or on $LD = 2:1$ (Aschoff et al., 1971). The authors believe that social cues dominate the pattern: but the possible influence of the regularity of the sampling procedure should not be overlooked (cf. p. 63).

Cellular effects

The study of circadian patterns in behaviour and macro-physiology has been accompanied by detailed micro-analytical investigations along various paths. As the cell is a fundamental biological unit, Bruce (1965) sought an answer to the question of whether the processes of cell division may not perhaps be governed by a diurnal rhythm. The basic DNA is synthesized in the first time interval or S phase which is preceded and followed by gaps G1 and G2 respectively. The fourth or M-phase intervenes between G2 and G1. M stands for mitosis, the process of physical cell division. Now the relative durations of these intervals vary in different cell types. But it can hardly be a matter of coincidence that the overall generation times of cells as different as chick skeletal muscle fibroblasts, pig kidney cells, and others are of the order of 24 h. Mitotic rhythms are especially marked in the epidermis which, like the retina, is derived embryologically from ectoderm. As the epidermis absorbs particularly u.v. radiation of wavelength 270 nm which shows a marked diurnal rhythm, obvious but as yet unexplored avenues of research open up. Now Bruce stresses that there are significant differences between the various mitotic peak times: e.g. in the mouse hepatic and epidermal mitoses peak in the middle of the day, whereas in the adrenal.cortex and parenchyma they do so in the middle of the night. That hormonal agents may be involved follows from the observations that, after nine days of time inversion, there is a corresponding phase change in the rhythms of liver parenchyma but not in the epidermal rhythm: it is as though the epidermal cell had a longer racial memory than is true of the parenchymatous one.

Again, if the liver tissue has been injured and starts to regenerate, the rhythm is set up by the moment of the injury operation. But the coupling between cell cycles is loose and therefore the circadian rhythm is loose. It would appear that the generalized cell, if this Goethean principle may be applied, possesses potentially, or in fact, many cyclic regulatory mechanisms with different periods. In addition, mutual interactions, or 'coupling strengths', may differ.

At a level more highly organized than can be true of individual cells, diurnal rhythms are also detected. For example the white corpuscles (leucocytes) of rat blood show a well-marked rhythm in the fluorescence of smears treated by the method which depends on intense greenish-yellow fluorescence being produced when the amines in a dried protein film are exposed to formaldehyde vapour: only those that are both primary and have OH-groups at the 3 and 4 positions (such as dopamine and noradrenaline) can be detected in this manner. When the animals were in the light from 08.00–20.00 hours, the smears fluoresced appreciably at 02.00 and 14.00 hours. In continuous illumination the rhythm was virtually abolished. No similar datum is available for human leucocytes, but it is claimed that fluorescence is more intense in male than in female cells, and there is evidence to suggest that it is higher in schizophrenia that in mental stability.

However, significant diurnal periodicity can be demonstrated even in isolated neurones. An electrode was inserted into an isolated suitably perfused and maintained, ganglion of the sea-hare *Aplysia californica*. After the animal had been subjected to a regime of nine cycles of light followed by darkness (LD = 12/12) impalement of the cell was continued for 48 h. Spontaneous peak activity was recorded first soon after the time when a light period would have occurred if the regime had gone on beyond No. 9. A second bout of enhanced activity occurred but with a delay of approximately 3 h. The amplitude was, however, reduced as though the expectation or, rather, the memory of the ganglion were fading (Fig. 2.9). In another neurone the delay (4 h) and reduction in amplitude were accentuated: the impalement had lasted 39 h and the integrity of the preparation may have been in doubt. The ratio of the amplitude of the second day to that of the first day after 'conditioning' had terminated fell with the length of the conditioning period; two days turned out to be insufficient for the memory to be revealed, three providing threshold stimulation which was evidently

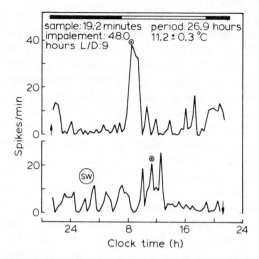

Fig. 2.9 Spike output of a single neurone as a function of clock time. The organism had been conditioned to nine cycles of light followed by darkness (L/D: 9). The second day of intracellular recording is plotted below the first. Period of dark and light (during past conditioning) indicated as shaded and clear portions, respectively, of the upper rectangular bar. 'Sample' refers to the successive lengths of time over which spikes were counted. 'Period' refers to the span of time between the two markers ($\odot$). At $\uparrow$ cell was impaled. Temperature indicated is the average followed by the range. Sea water (SW) changed in main reservoir at zero hours. (After Strumwasser, 1965.)

cumulative. When a ganglion was used from an animal that had been kept in constant illumination for seven days, the 'free-run' period elapsing before the activity peaked was only 21 h. When pre-illumination went on for ten days, the period rose to 25 h. Strumwasser was able to demonstrate also the existence of a semi-lunar cycle (14 d). The origin of these rhythms is, in all probability, endogenous as there is no evidence of any appropriate pigment (though effects due to short wavelength radiation have not been ruled out, cf. p. 72), and the circadian burst fails to be suppressed even with hyperpolarization strong enough to eliminate all background activity.

Synchronization

While it is evident that very different types of tissue can exhibit circadian rhythms and that these may be endogenous, memorized, or both, this situation exists as it were at the molecular level. It leaves out of account the important problem of synchronization. From the point of view of biology, there are two principal mechanisms one of which is subdivided as shown in the following summary:

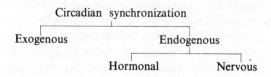

Exogenous synchronization presupposes an animal with a large surface/volume ratio: in practice this means animals that are so small that virtually all their tissues can be simultaneously affected by light, temperature etc. Since a high water content offers a means for stabilizing temperature, vertebrate species which consist to over 90 per cent of water are not readily accommodated in this group: the fact that the water content of insects can be as low as 50 per cent is worthy of note. But vertebrates have developed endogenous methods, i.e. a primitive and a phylogenetically more recent one for maintaining tissue control methods which can be compared with sending messages by hand (hormonal) and by radio (nervous) respectively.

In this context we ought to remind ourselves that, by and large, the body is not in a great hurry to be informed of regular changes in the external environment. Let us for the moment disregard the cellular and subcellular clocks mentioned on the previous pages. Environmental changes occur slowly as compared with an animal's ability to move e.g. from light into shade and *vice versa*. The time constants of circadian rhythms have therefore to be long if metabolic waste is to be minimized. It follows that the flow of blood may have a rate of movement which meets this purpose; that specialized organs sensitive to circadian changes may alter the composition of blood in such a manner as to inform relatively distant tissues that it is time to go to sleep, to recharge batteries, to get rid of waste products, to regenerate cells that are exhausted etc. We ought to remind ourselves also that the rate of dark-adaptation which changes the sensitivity of the human eye from a level adequate for daylight vision to one enabling it to perform optimally at minimum levels of illumination (Fig. 2.10) does so in the course of some 30–40 minutes. This is commensurate not only with some sort of approximation to homeostasis which is desirable on perceptual grounds (cf. eq. 2.2 on p. 59) but also with the rate with which circadian effects due to light build up and fall off.

Dark-adaptation as a circadian problem

At this point it may be legitimately objected that a major part of the sensitivity gain manifested as dark-adaptation is neural in origin and that, insofar as ionic transport is involved in this, this is not mediated by the blood-stream, and occurs, in any case, over synaptic distances which are smaller by several orders of magnitude than is true of the inter-tissue paths mentioned above. However, this is an argument based on hind-sight. Nervous messages are carried from tissue to tissue at speeds very much greater than is true of the blood-stream. For example a nervous discharge can travel along fibres of the spinal chord with a velocity of up to 120 m/s whereas the rate of blood-flow never exceeds 0.5 m/s. The type of control exercised by hormones and by nervous messages is distinguished not only by their relative velocities but also by their *modi operandi*: the hormone is the agent, the nervous message a word of command. In the former case execution does not need any intervening agent, in the latter.it does.

It is not so much the rapidity of nervous conduction that is to be wondered at, as the slowness of dark-adaptation. One asks oneself whether there has been any evolutionary pressure to promote a rate of adaptation to darkness appreciably greater than that of loss of light due to the setting sun. The answer is clearly No.

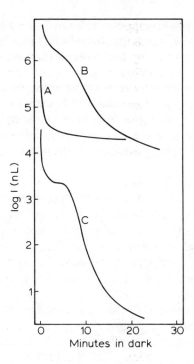

Fig. 2.10 Dark-adaptation curves obtained under three conditions (cf. Fig. 2.16 below). A: the foveal centre (test diameter d ~ 3′); B: 8° in the left nasal visual field (d ~ 3′); C: 8° in the left nasal field (d ~ 7°). Note the similarity between the final thresholds in A and B, and the difference in the rates at which the final rod thresholds are reached in B and C. This is an example of different rates of neuronal coupling changes as revealed by large and small fields respectively. (After Arden and Weale, 1954.)

At the same time, one faces the question whether there has been any evolutionary pressure against an acceleration in dark-adaptation. If dark-adaptation proceeded very much faster than it does, i.e. if a reduction in intensity caused a rapid rise in sensitivity to the (weaker) stimuli reaching the eye, their apparent brightness could well be greater than that of the earlier stronger stimuli. The synchronizing function of dusk would consequently become complicated if in no other sense than that the photic signals received by the eye could become operationally ambiguous, and the time of action available to it would be correspondingly shortened. The tentative hypothesis to advance is therefore that the rate of dark adaptation has been reached by an evolutionary pressure striving to match it to the duration of the onset of the falling-off of such circadian rhythms as happen to occur at or near sunset and are under photic control.

Hormonal control–lower animals

The hormonal control of circadian rhythms is a subject of widespread studies, and complicated by the mutual interaction between various glands. As is well-known, the adrenal glands are under pituitary control: the adreno-corticotropic hormone secreted by the adreno-hypophysis or the anterior lobe of the pituitary gland exerts an indirect control on muscle tone by virtue of its effect on adrenal secretion. Since, as we shall see below, the pituitary glands of many animals are influenced by light, it is not hard to see a causal nexus in the chain of darkness-sleep-muscle relaxation.

It is important to stress this link as, in many animals, the photic influence on the pituitary manifests largely at the gonadal level. In man (Fig. 2.11), the gland lies so deeply embedded in the head that it is hard to remember that it represents phylogenetically the homologue of an organ that is light-sensitive, e.g. in the frog, as is true of the so-called third eye, or stirnorgan (p. 74).

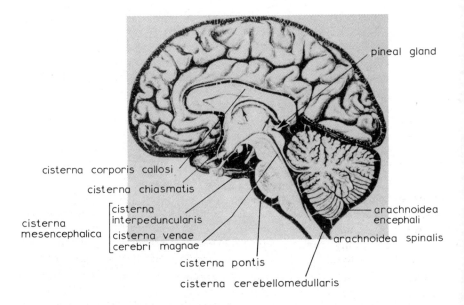

Fig. 2.11   Topography of the pineal gland (P) in man. The arrows indicate the position of the velum interpositum which is rich in cerebral veins. (After Kappers, 1976.)

The pineal gland has a recent history as regards our understanding of its chemistry (Kappers, 1976). It contains several biogenic amines such as catecholamines and indoleamines which figure frequently as indices of circadian activity (cf. p. 67). Their presence is detected by the Flack-Hillarp fluorescence technique mentioned in connection with diurnal rhythms in leucocytes (cf. p. 68). One of the most important indole compounds to be found in the gland (Fig. 2.12) is serotonin, the injection of which into even as relatively low an animal as *Aplysia*, modifies the circadian rhythm. One of the intervening compounds, namely N-acetyl-5-methoxytryptamine or melatonin causes the aggregation of the pigment granules in frog skin (whence its name): as frogs tend to mimic their environment, the photic involvement of the pituitary is readily manifested in this camouflage.

The removal of the pineal gland has not always yielded unequivocal results, and the age of the operated individual animal plays an important role. The main effects appear in the gonads. But whereas female hormones, such as oestrogen

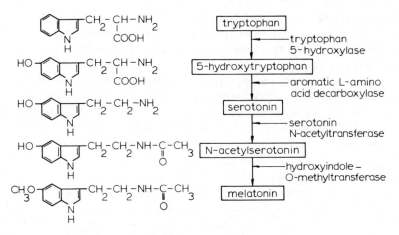

Fig. 2.12 Biosynthesis of melatonin from tryptophan in the pineal gland. (After Kappers, 1976.)

and progesterone, if given to males in large doses, lead to an enlargement of the mammary glands and even to lactation, this does not occur in hypophysectomized animals. This suggests that the above steroids act on the pituitary and the effect of light which induces oestrus e.g. in hamsters and ferrets is to modify this action (cf. below). Another pituitary hormone, namely prolactin, also manifests a diurnal cycle in its blood concentration, as we shall detail in a moment, and we must not forget the posterior lobe or the neurohypophysis which exerts control e.g. over body temperature.

More significantly from our point of view, the pituitary is under nervous control from the hypothalamus which may mediate photic control and does so definitely in the anoestrous ferret being brought in midwinter into oestrus by prolonged exposure to light. In the rat, extending the L/D ratio from normal to greater values up to infinity leads to an increase in the weight of the ovaries and to precocious oestrus. This is accompanied by a reduction in the content of pineal serotonin. The latter acts as an inhibitor. Prolonged darkness (and blindness) produce opposite effects; and generally promote pineal activity. There are, however, important species variations: the hamster provides an example of the pineal organ exerting maximum antigonadotrophic activity. In many cases, the active substance is melatonin, though, as we saw above, its precursors can act by being converted into it if the requisite enzymes are present.

The action of pineal antigonadotrophic factors appears to take place in the hypothalamus, although the gonads themselves have also been implicated. It is not clear how the effect of light differs in the two cases (but see below). There is a well-authenticated circadian rhythm in the pineal serotonin content in the rat: a peak is reached during the middle of the day. In this context it is noteworthy that with melatonin injected into young adult rats 8 h after the onset of a photoperiod (LD = 14:10) the circadian rhythm in 5-hydroxytryptamine (or serotonin) is abolished, whereas at the end of the light phase it is ineffective. Serotonin has been implicated in the neural control of circadian rhythms, and shows high concentrations in the pineal gland at the beginning of the L phase when LD = 8:16.

There is little diurnal change when LD = 14:10. A very different picture prevails in the hypothalamus: the pineal variation appears here at a much lower amplitude when LD is low. When LD is high the hypothalamus presents a mirror image of the pituitary situation for low LD values. It remains to be decided to what extent the circadian rhythm of serotonin may be governed by a diurnal variation in the release of the neurotransmitter noradrenaline, present in the pineal sympathetic nerves. They release more of this substance nocturnally than during the day: here we may not be concerned with a photic effect so much as one due for example to the sleep cycle.

The actual control on the serotonin pathway appears to be exerted photically on enzymes facilitating the transformation (Fig. 2.12). The key roles are played by serotonin N-acetyltransferase which converts serotonin to N-acetylserotonin, and hydroxyindole-O-methyltransferase which synthesizes melatonin from the latter.

It is worth stressing on phylogenetic grounds that in many sub-mammalian vertebrate such as batracians (frogs, toads), and lizards, the stirnorgan responds to light even when the lateral eyes are removed. It possesses structures morphologically and photophysiologically similar to retinal photo-receptors. On the other hand, in the adult mammal neural intervention is needed.

Hormonal effects—man

The afore-mentioned species differences obviously make it impossible to extend the above observations to man without adequate experimental evidence. Some of them would not be expected: e.g. the oestrous cycle is not an annual event as in the ferret or hamster. Nevertheless, the existence of well-marked behavioural and physiological circadian rhythms in man necessitates a search for hormonal and neural causes. Osterman and Wide (1975) studied the concentration of plasma prolactin in three males and one nulliparous female (as motherhood changes the situation). Prolactin is a hormone formed in the anterior pituitary gland: as far as is known its formation is independent of effects due to other pituitary hormones. A diurnal rhythm having been established earlier, the authors wondered whether this was due to the sleep or the LD pattern. The experimental arrangement involved a constant sleep-waking cycle (8:16). During a control period of ten days lighting followed the same pattern, but during another ten days the LD ratio was changed to 12:12. The results show that the average prolactin was higher during the control periods than during the periods with prolonged darkness, though no level of statistical significance is given. This agrees essentially with less well-controlled experiments on animals.

Modern studies on man involve assays obtained from catheters inserted e.g. into the antecubital vein (on the inside of the elbow) or from urine analysis. Interpretations of alleged photic and other effects have to be circumspect. While a substance present in blood plasma at any time *may* be there for use rather than because it is no longer used, this cannot be true of urinary contents. Such re-absorption as occurs in the renal tubules recycles what can be retrieved and what is left in urine is lost to the body. Consequently cyclic changes in urinary contents may be a reflection of diurnal variations in absorption, which, in turn, may arise from cycles in metabolic demand. It follows that diurnal peak concentrations in urine may point to periods of minimal systemic use, i.e. it cannot be taken for granted that a positive correlation with other circadian rhythms is of significance let alone potentially in causal relation.

Although it may be difficult for the above reasons to establish valid causal connections between photic influences and circadian rhythms in any one individual, there is, unfortunately, a ready-made line of attack available to us by comparing blind with sighted subjects. For example the secretion of cortisol (from the adrenal glands) was found to be circadian in five out of seven blind subjects (Weitzman, 1976). The observation was made that members of the Norwegian Air Force, stationed above the Arctic Circle, maintained a constant circadian pattern in cortisol secretion even though there was a seasonal variation in the mean daily plasma concentration; but this study was not fully controlled. On balance, however, the circadian cortisol rhythm does not appear to be under photic control. This conclusion is reinforced by a study on one male and one female adult when plasma cortisol (11-OHCS, see below) levels, urinary volume, Na^+, K^+, Cl^-, and creatinine were sampled every four hours, the subjects sleeping in the dark from 0 until 08.00 hours and pursuing 'usual daily activities' for 48 hours. The regime was then repeated after 21 days of zero darkness (with no mention being made of light transmitted by the eye-lids during sleep) and again following a subsequent 13-day period of zero darkness, but the sleep-wake cycle changed to sleep from noon to 20.00 hours. The data indicate that the cortisol cycle and also the variation in urinary electrolytes is governed by the sleep-wake synchronizer and not by light (Fig. 2.13).

The secretion of [pituitary] growth hormone was found to be sleep-related in five out of seven blind subjects (Weitzman, 1976), but as blind people may have abnormal sleep patterns, further work is needed before a convincing comparison can be made with normal data.

Positive evidence that light does play a role in human endocrine activity was obtained (well before Weitzman's penetrating review) by Orth and Island who

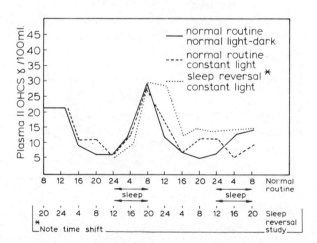

Fig. 2.13 Circadian pattern of plasma (11-OHCS) cortisol levels under 3 different regimens of sleep-activity, light-dark. (From Krieger, Kreuzer and Rizzo, 1969. © J. B. Lippincott Co., Philadelphia.)

examined hourly samples of blood for 17,21-dihydroxy-20-ketosteroids (17-OHCS) obtained from the distal forearm vein. They kept five normal subjects on a strict sleep-wake cycle (8:12) in a light-proof suite of rooms, and imposed three experimental LD schedules. In the first, 8 h of total darkness started 12 h after the onset of sleep. In the second, darkness continued for 4 h after waking up. The third involved continuous darkness except for 1 h of light from 18.00 to 19.00 hours. Three totally blind persons were also studied. The conclusions to be drawn from this study – which are not necessarily those drawn by the authors – are (a) that light reduces the level of 17-OHCS to a greater extent than does waking, and (b) that blind men exhibit the 'waking' moiety of the normal circadian rhythm. The inevitable scatter of the data and the absence of a statistical evaluation make it difficult to enter with confidence into a discussion of other interesting points raised by this study.

Although, therefore, light affects man in ways other than those expected merely on the basis of the ingestion and digestion of information, it is still undecided whether the effect is profound. For example, workers who have been 13 weeks on night shifts have a distorted rather than a reversed temperature rhythm (Fig. 2.14). On the other hand, as many of us know, jet-lag takes up to five days to overcome. In fact, westward travel is easier to take than is true of the opposite. The reason appears to be that when our circadian rhythms are on a free-run they tend to a 25 h day (cf. pp. 65–67) and in westward travel at least one day is lengthened: westward flights are physiologically shorter than eastward ones. Both in shift work and in international travel, the changes in the light-dark pattern are accompanied by one in the sleep-wake rhythm. Since a night shift usually implies starting work before midnight, the situation is equivalent to an extended day (cf. westward flight), and the protracted deformation of the temperature pattern is, at

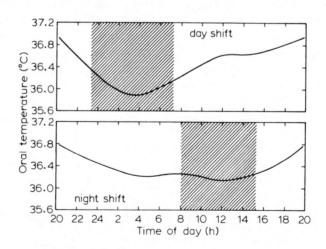

Fig. 2.14 The effect of shift time on body temperature rhythms was recorded in three males who were studied while working day shifts and again after 13 weeks of working nights. Workers on night shifts show a temperature drop about half that of day workers, indicating a deformation of rhythm rather than a complete phase reversal. (After Aschoff, 1976.)

best, puzzling: no such prolonged hysteresis was observed in temperature measurements after simulated interzonal flights when the temperature rhythm was fully adjusted within 11–12 days after flying west, and 14–15 after flights in the opposite direction. It is significant that the L/D and W/S patterns are concordant in the jet situation but at odds when night shifts are involved. It may well be that the relatively weak photic chronodon can play a role in short-term disturbances but not in prolonged ones. Analogous tests on blind volunteers might well produce a conclusive solution.

Circadianism and vision

If there are circadian rhythms immediately based on light, and others, as it were, remember being conditioned by it a multitude of generations ago, then it is natural to ask oneself whether the very instrument whereby the rhythms may have been established – namely eyes with their nervous paraphernalia – do not also take part in this circadian round. This possibility is implicit in the argument presented on p. 59. If we look on the afferent and efferent parts of the nervous assembly from the point of view of systems analysis then we can compare the physics of circadian rhythms with an input/output situation. The rhythms are that which manifests. The issue is whether the input is circadian or whether perhaps the sensitivity of the black box between the input and output is periodic. A study of the input or output alone may be inconclusive: we need to know the transfer characteristics of the system. Here we are faced with remarkable gaps in our knowledge.

It is plainly inadmissible to answer questions about visual circadianism by means of animal behaviour experiments. In man, the situation is somewhat simpler because he can communicate the results of introspection. Thus the decision whether or not a stimulus of a given intensity was seen does not involve behaviour in the same sense in which a cat may be trained to move to the left when it has seen the light and to the right when it has not done so. Strangely enough, the number of experiments to have tested circadianism in man can apparently be counted on the fingers of one hand. Part of the explanation of this curious state of affairs is that such experiments, even short-term ones tend to be dreary: to try and persuade people to submit to such tests at regular or irregular intervals during one or more 24 hour cycles is enough to test any friendship or professional relationship.

Harper and Zubek (1976) determined the critical flicker or fusion frequency (i.e. that frequency at which the illumination due to a variably intermittent stimulus just appears continuous) in 36 university students. These volunteers agreed to wear a blindfold over both eyes for a whole week. One group wore an opaque mask while another wore a diffusing one, which acted like a fog, admitting into the eyes light but no contour. One control group was used. The fusion frequency was measured every three hours during the first day (except after 18 hours) and then once every day till the third; after this once every other day. The fusion frequency showed no variation in any of the three groups although the general circadian rhythms must have been disturbed at least in the group with the opaque masks. Note that, in this test, the question of circadianism did not arise: nor was it considered.

Reaction-time, a quantity beloved by experimental psychologists as a criterion of e.g. psychomotor performance, has been studied by several authors as an index of circadianism. Thus Aschoff (1976) reports that it reaches a minimum in the afternoon at 15.00 hours and rises to a maximum of surprising magnitude (> 550ms) at 03.00 in the morning (Fig. 2.15). Its variation offers therefore almost a mirror image to that of the rectal temperature. Superficially, this relation may not be surprising: nervous conduction time is faster at high than at low temperatures. But the amplitude of this variation (6 per cent) is too large to be explained simply in terms of temperature, and a smaller amplitude would probably not have been statistically significant: Aschoff quotes no variance for the dark. A smaller variation (±4 per cent) is reported by Knoerchen and Hildebrandt (1976); it showed a similar circadian course.

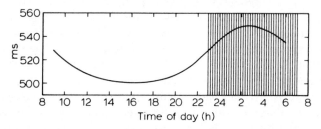

Fig. 2.15   Optical reaction time as a function of time of day. (After Aschoff, 1976.)

These authors made the first really extensive investigation into the diurnal variation of some of the visual capabilities of man though in 1951 Bornschein had measured in six persons absolute visual thresholds at 07.00, 11.00 and 18.00 hours and found a small but statistically significant peak in the middle measurement. This brilliant study stands in stark contrast with the more recent one, marred by inadequate controls and a fundamental misunderstanding of basic visual processes. The authors studied visual functions in subjects kept on a regime of 8 h darkness followed by 4 h of light (500 lux; 1 lx = 1 lm/sq m, cf. p. 5). In another series subjects were tested every 3 h and stayed in bed in complete darkness in between tests. Although both experiment and interpretation leave a great deal to be desired, the uniqueness of the study and the lessons to be learnt from its shortcomings make it worthy of a more detailed analysis than its quality might otherwise justify.

In addition to the above-mentioned measurements of the reaction time, tests were done on dark-adaptation following a 10 min exposure to a source of 3000 lux (cf. Fig. 2.10). No fixation point was used: in other words, there is no indication as to which part of the retina was being tested at any one time. In view of the non-uniform sensitivity of the retina both in its light- and dark-adapted states, this grave omission unnecessarily increased the variance of the data, on which no information is given. The processing of the data, e.g. the summation of thresholds measured during every one of 30 minutes of dark-adaptation, is meaningless as the early part of the curve relates to the more rapid adaptation of the cone-mechanism while the later part describes the slower processes of the rod-mechanism (see below). This division of the two curves is well understood: it reflects the duplex nature of the human visual system with the cone mechanism dominating diurnal vision, whereas the rods act principally at low levels of illumination.

There is a vague discontinuity between the two parts of the curve (cf. Figs. 2.10, 2.16). In the German literature it is held to be abrupt and referred to as the α-point, following Kohlrausch who first observed it in 1922. But it is easy to see that, even on theoretical grounds, a sharp transition is unlikely. In the neighbourhood of this point, the thresholds of the rod- and cone-mechanisms are approximately equal. But this means that, over a finite time-interval, the visual impulse can be initiated, with equal probability, by one or the other system even if no neural interaction occurs between them. Consequently a discontinuity such as that indicated above and used as a criterion also by US workers can be dismissed as improbable both on theoretical and on experimental grounds. Knoerchen and Hildebrandt, more confident in the precision of their data than inspection of same seems to merit, claim that there is a diurnal variation of this point: it appears earliest in the dark-adaptation curve when this is measured at 22.00 hours and later when the measurements are done in the afternoon at 15.00 hours. What does this mean?

The dark-adaptation curve can be considered as the envelope of at least two curves: namely a cone and a rod mechanism curve as shown schematically in Fig. 2.16. If the α-point appears earlier than usual the cone curve must be higher in relation to the rod curve and *vice versa*. It follows that, if valid, this result of Knoerchen and Hildebrandt's demonstrates different diurnal variations for the

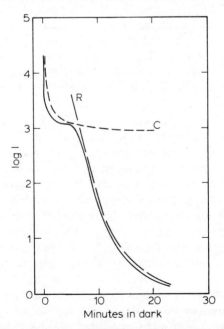

Fig. 2.16 The analysis of a bimodal dark-adaptation curve into components governed by different neural mechanisms (cf. Fig. 2.10). In this instance external evidence points to the early part representing the dark-adaptation of cone mechanisms (not just cones), and the later that of rod mechanisms (not just rods).

two mechanisms, a vital point that has apparently escaped them. It does not, however, rule out the possibility that, in one or the other, the variation is zero, but the two variations cannot be the same contrary to the implication made by the authors' summation of the data.

Some little progress can be made e.g. by a consideration of the thresholds during the first and last four minutes. In all probability these relate purely to the cone and rod thresholds respectively. The authors give values with up to six significant places: it is, however, better to use logarithms, and the logged averages of the above four sets of measurements are shown in Fig. 2.17a. They are consistent with an early time for the α-point at approximately 22.00 hours. But when we consider the variability of the results by comparing the first and last values (at 09.00 hours) then this consistency is not firmly based. One should hasten to add that an experimental error of 0.1 log units is not excessive. But what is needed here is a statistical analysis telling us the probability that the shapes of the two curves (as distinct from their absolute values) differ by more than chance.

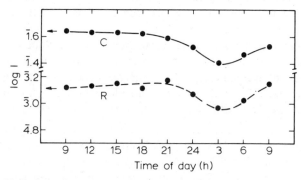

Fig. 2.17a   Variation of cone (C) and rod (R) thresholds during 24 hours when the pupillary diameter is not controlled. (Based on data from Knoerchen and Hildebrandt, 1976.)

The data in Fig. 2.17a suggest that both rods and cones reach their minimum thresholds at about 03.00 hours in the morning. In view of the data discussed on p. 91 this is a matter of considerable interest. Parallel tests involved the lowest intensity at which the observers could identify the position of the gap in a Landolt C corresponding to a visual acuity of 0.05, i.e. one twentieth normal. This corresponds to a spatial frequency of 3c/° and is easily resolved by the rod mechanism at low luminance levels (cf. Ch. 1). It is not surprising, therefore, that these results closely follow those shown in Fig. 2.17a. Both the Landolt C data and those on p. 78 are threshold measurements, differing only in the criterion adopted to determine a critical stimulus intensity: 'seeing a gap' in one case and 'seeing light' in the other.

Knoerchen and Hildebrandt's observations throw interesting light on a study of the circadian rhythms of the pupil area (Döring and Schaefers, 1950). These authors measured the pupil diameter entoptically by placing two small apertures at a variable distance in the anterior focal planes of the eyes of their six (young) observers. Each aperture gave rise to a circular retinal image outlining the pupil. When the separation between the two apertures equalled the pupillary diameter the two circular images just touched. This measurement was done ten times every three hours, care being taken to keep the light intensity constant. Fig. 2.17b shows that on average, the pupillary area varied by about 45 per cent between a minimum in the early and a maximum in the late morning. The authors conclude that this demonstrates a circadian rhythm in the size of the pupil. In view of the (later) results of Fig. 2.17a this conclusion needs special attention. Owing to the light reflex, the diameter of the pupil varies inversely with retinal illuminance. Thus when the threshold is at its lowest, the sensitivity of the eye will tend to constrict the pupil (cf. p. 59) even if the physical light intensity is kept constant.

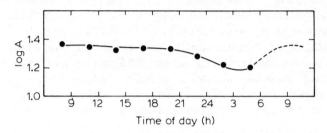

Fig. 2.17b Variation of pupillary area during 24 hours. (After Döring and Schaefers, 1950.)

Hence keeping the light intensity constant involved the wrong control: what should have been kept constant is the intensity expressed in threshold units. It is possible that attention to this point might have reduced the apparent variation in pupillary diameter, but unlikely that it would have eliminated it altogether since the intensity needed to elicit the pupil reflex is relatively high. Conversely, a change in retinal illuminance R can result from a small change in pupil diameter. As the data in Fig. 2.17a were obtained without a small artificial pupil, and the natural pupil was at its smallest when threshold was at its lowest, the true circadian variation of the threshold I has to be determined from the relation $I = R/A$ where A is the pupillary area in sq mm. Note that this correction (Fig. 2.17a) accentuates the drop in the original intensity measurements at 05.00 hours.

The above criticisms are made emphatically so that they may perhaps encourage the student of visual science who has expertise in this field to venture into the important aspects of circadianism on which the above authors have shed useful light. The matter has become more urgent as a result of a number of some startling observations made by several American researchers on vertebrate photo-receptors.

The retina under circadian influence

Phylogenetically the eye or, more accurately, the retina represents photo-sensitive dermis; and, indeed, even on an embryological basis it is derived from neural ectoderm. Nervous tissue is laid down by cell-division once and for all: if this were not the case it is hard to see how memory could develop and be maintained. The photo-receptors are part of the retina and, until a few years ago, were believed to be likewise laid down for life. Indeed, Young, who has greatly contributed to our present-day understanding of receptor formation, believed as recently as 1971 that the cones owe their shape to the fact that their tips are their oldest part, formed when the retina was young and therefore small. He thought that the maintenance of this shape in the face of the cylindrical form of rods which had been shown to go on regenerating in periods not exceeding a few weeks in duration in all species examined (Young, 1967) was due to the permanence of the cones. This view has been supplanted in the light of more recent evidence mentioned below. As receptor renewal is subject to circadian rhythms, it falls within the purview of our inquiry, and a brief account of the relevant method of investigation may be of interest.

The investigations were based on the technique of autoradiography. If radio-active amino-acids are supplied to an animal they are incorporated into certain protein molecules if these are renewed. If sections are cut from tissues so impregnated each decaying radio-active atom exposes a silver halide grain once the section is brought into juxtaposition with a photographic emulsion. Young supplied such traces to a number of animals, which were sacrificed at various intervals after the ingestion of the amino-acids. In the case of rods, it turned out that, while the newly synthesized protein concentrates near the boundary

Fig. 2.18 Radio-autograms depicting rods and cones, 2 and 4 days after injection of leucine-^{3}H. The pigment epithelium is visible at the top of each photograph. $0.5\,\mu$ sections, stained with toluidine blue. Bar $= 10\,\mu$.
A Two days after injection of leucine-^{3}H, a transverse band of radioactive protein (upper arrow) is present near the base (lower arrow) of each rod outer segment. By contrast, no such concentration of radioactivity appears in the outer segment of the cone (c, far left). pe, pigment epithelium; is, rod inner segments.
B The outer segments of two cones are visible (arrows). Both contain newly formed, radio-active protein, which is not, however, localized as in the rods, 2 days after injection. The scattered, relatively weak radio-autographic reaction is comparable to that present in the outer part of the rod outer segments. In both instances newly formed protein has penetrated the pre-existing disc structure.
C The zone of concentrated labeled protein near the base of each rod is considered to be due to a group of intensely labeled discs formed immediately after the injection, 2 days earlier, and now displaced partly along the outer segment as a result of continued disc formation. There is no evidence of new disc assembly in the cone (arrow).
D The radio-active discs have been displaced a similar distance from the base in each rod, indicating comparable rates of disc production. The three cone outer segments (arrows) contain relatively small amounts of diffusely distributed new protein.
E The radio-autograms reveal that the process of outer segment renewal differs in rods and cones. Labeling is weak and diffuse in the cone outer segment (arrow) and in the outer part of the rod outer segments (x). The discs near the base of the rod outer segments are heavily labeled because they were assembled during the 2 days since the injection of radioactive leucine.
F Two days after injection, newly formed, intensely radio-active discs (middle arrow) have been displaced a short distance from the base (lower arrow) of the rod outer segment. By measuring that distance, and the length of the rod outer segment (distance between upper and lower arrows), it is possible to estimate the rod outer segment renewal time. This proved to range between 9 and 13 days in different parts of the retina.
G Four days after injection, the intensely radioactive discs (middle arrow) have been further displaced. They are now situated approximately halfway between the base (lower arrow) and the extremity (upper arrow) of the outer segment. The rods in (F) are from the parafovea; those in (G) are from the periphery of the retina. Note that the rod outer segments are shorter in the periphery. (From Young, 1971b. © The Rockefeller University Press, New York.)

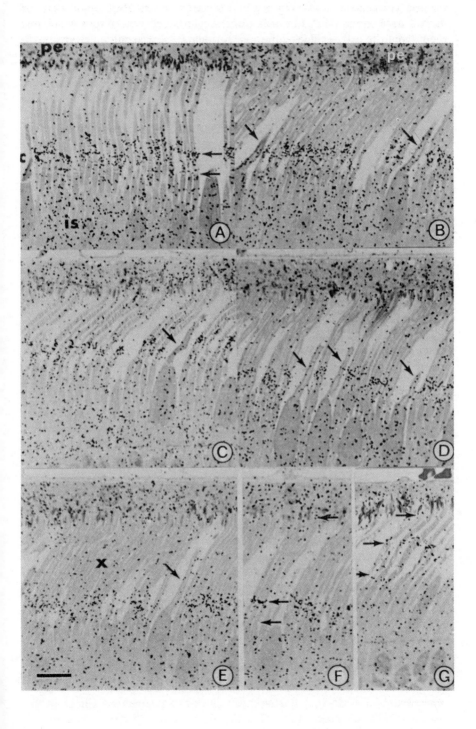

between the inner and the outer limbs, a significant portion of the radio-active material forms date-bands. When we recall that rods are made up of stacks of individual twin-disks (Fig. 1.20) that are contained in a surrounding sac insulating them from the extra-cellular environment, then it is reasonable to explain the apico-petal movement of the date-bands in terms of a gradual displacement of the individual lamellae away from the inner limb toward the tip of the rod.

If this formation of lamellae were continual, the rods would increase in length with results for the intactness of the retina that are not hard to divine. In view of our earlier emphasis on the ectodermal origin of the neural retina, the membrane renewal of the photo-receptors cannot come altogether as a surprise: the mechanism is related to that of the continual growth of the crystalline lens, the continuous growth of nails, hair and the formation of the skin. But what is unique is the disposal of the surplus lamellae. The structure near the tip weakens periodically (cf. p. 22), till lamellar segments break away to be devoured or phagocytozed by the processes of the retinal pigment epithelium that envelop the receptor tips.

No such situation can be observed in cones (Fig. 2.18). The radio-active material appears to suffuse them unbanded. The cones, too, exhibit a lamellar structure. However, as distinct from that of the rods, the enveloping membrane is continuous with the lamellar folds, forming with them a single sheet which offers little let or hindrance to the relatively small molecules (Fig. 2.18): these can therefore travel rapidly throughout the whole cone structure. Thus, while both rod and cone outer limbs can be labelled, morphological constraints impose literally a date-line on the former but not on the latter.

The cone membrane is, however, no less impermanent than that of the rods. Even human cone membranes are shed in a manner similar to that observed for primate rods, and the debris is phagocytozed by the phagosomes of the retinal pigment epithelium. Anderson *et al.* (1978) showed in fact on the basis of studies of cones from the retinae of squirrels, cats, monkeys and man that rods and cones fare similarly: they experience a complete turnover made up essentially of a balanced formation of lamellae near the base of the outer limb and ultimate apical fragmentation followed by phagocytosis by the processes of the retinal pigment epithelium.

This observation has an important corollary. It implies that this renewal of the outer limbs may represent a type of repair mechanism. Clinically, it has been known for decades that a solar burn accompanied as it is by a scotoma or blind spot, need not herald permanent destruction of the overexposed receptors. It is significant from our point of view that 'in general, it may be said that the prognosis will probably be good if the symptoms, particularly the scotoma, subside during the first month'. Foveal visual acuity has been known to be fully restored weeks or months after accidental photic overexposure. As this is, unfortunately, not the inevitable rule, one can only surmise that trauma to the inner limb causes irreparable damage, while if the disturbance is confined to the lamellar part of the photo-receptor, the normal process of renewal may restore function. This explanation is inadequate because renewal is completed at intervals lasting weeks to a few months: for example, cone outer limbs in the rhesus retina have a renewal period lasting from 8.8 to 12.8 days depending on retinal location: the more peripheral they are the more quickly they regenerate

(Young, 1971b). These times are commensurate with those observed e.g. for rat and mouse rods (Young, 1967). Returning to retinal damage: longer periods of recovery are at present unexplained. But the above hypothesis also makes it harder to attribute senile cell death (cf. Ch. 3) to a cumulative effect of light damage in the photo-receptor outer limbs.

Young's elegant studies left, however, one uncomfortable impression: it looked as though there were some species in which cones did not regenerate. This led to more and more penetrating inquiries into the whole question of disk formation and shedding, and to the resolution of the problem in terms of circadianism. The significance of this conclusion would obviously have been harder to appreciate without acquaintance with some of the preceding detail. Moreover, by an ironic quirk, a problem relating to the cones was solved by observations done on rods.

In a study of the rat retina, La Vail (1976) examined disk shedding in relation to the lighting cycle. He kept inbred Fischer albino rats in a controlled photic environment with fluorescent light on at 07.00 hours and off at 19.00 hours. The animals were sacrificed at various times of the 24 h cycle, and the retinae prepared for disk-phagosome counts. Phagosomes are bodies that take up toluidine blue and are larger than 0.75μ. They ingest shed receptor disks, and are found in the pigment epithelium cell somata and processes, although location in the latter site could be due to artifactual mechanical dislocation.

La Vail found that the number of large phagosomes varied with the phase of the lighting cycle. As seen in Fig. 2.19, it was maximal immediately after cessation of darkness. Since the rat is a nocturnal animal, this suggests that the pigment epithelium is ready to digest rods at a time when they are not of much use to the animal: but no one seems as yet to have followed up this observation e.g. with a study of the animal's electro-retinographic sensitivity throughout the day.

How much darkness is needed to elicit the sort of burst seen in Fig. 2.19a? Dark periods lasting less than about 12 h are ineffectual, but there seems to be some variability in these difficult counts. The question of whether light has a direct effect on the counts is answered by the experiment summarized in Fig. 2.19b. When rats were kept in the dark for up to three days, the biggest burst occurred at a time when light would have come on if the original régime had been maintained. It is plain that a rhythm had been entrained, and that the rods remembered it, much as we noticed with the ganglion of *Aplysia* (Fig. 2.8). At present, there is no indication as to the length of the memory, but there is little doubt that it is entrained by light.

However, this is not necessarily a universal property. For example when frogs, *Rana pipiens*, were kept on an artificial light regime (LD = 14:10), no shed phagosome was observed at the onset of light at 7.50 h (Fig. 2.20). An hour later the number rose to a sharp peak, and the rods that had shed their apices (some 25 per cent) appeared somewhat shorter than those that had not. If the frogs are kept in the dark after 7.50 h no new phagosome appears: in other words, the process is light-induced and not subject to a circadian rhythm, light-entrained or otherwise. However, some 'dark' shedding occurs together with phagocytosis, but on a non-synchronous basis. Also, after six days' darkness, the rod outer limbs are about 12 per cent longer than when the LD regime is maintained.

Besharse *et al.* (1977) looked at the other end of the process, albeit in a comparatively primitive eye. They injected *Rana pipiens* and *Xenopus laevis*

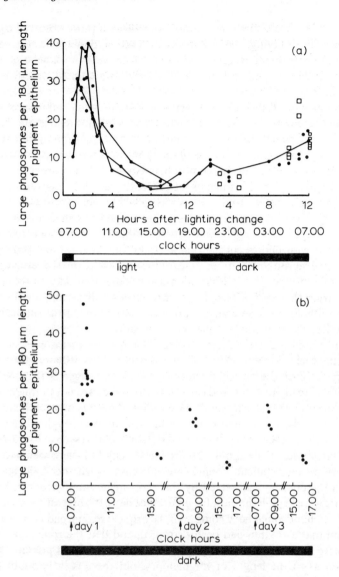

Fig. 2.19 Counts of large phagosomes at different times of the lighting cycle. Each point represents the mean number of phagosomes found in ten 180 μm lengths of pigment epithelium in the eye of a single rat; five consecutive 180 μm lengths were examined in the posterior part of the retina on each side of the optic nerve head with 100 $\times$ oil immersion optics. (a) Counts in cyclic lighting. The three curves represent separate experiments. The individual points represent additional animals perfused in other individual experiments. ($\square$): rats that were taken from the dark and placed in the light 1 hour before perfusion (perfusion time indicated by data). ($\bullet$) located 1 hour before ($\square$) represent control animals taken immediately from the dark in the same experiment as the animals represented by the following ($\square$); they were usually litter-mates. (b) Counts in continuous darkness. The arrows indicate when the lights would have come on if the rats had been in cyclic lighting. (From La Vail, 1976, © by the American Association for the Advancement of Science.)

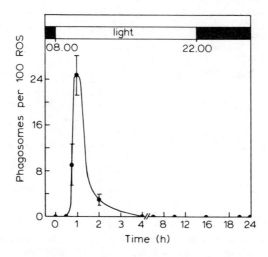

Fig 2.20 Time course of shedding of ROS (rod outer segments) in the frog retina. With well-oriented longitudinal sections taken from frogs at the indicated times (●) the number of newly shed phagosomes was counted and expressed as number of phagosomes per 100 ROS. Synchronous shedding is observed in about 25 per cent of the ROS within the first 2 hours of the diurnal cycle. The bar at the top shows the light and dark phases of the diurnal cycle (14 hours light and 10 hours darkness). (From Basinger, Hoffman and Matthes, 1976. © 1976 by the American Association for the Advancement of Science.)

tadpoles intraperitoneally with $25 \mu c$ of $[4,5-^3H]$ L-leucine, and for a week before, and one day after, the injection the animals were kept in LD = 12:12. Then some of the animals were sacrificed, while one group was kept for up to 12 days in LL, another in DD, a third in LD = 12:12, and a fourth in LD = 2:22. The positions of the radio-active band (cf. p. 84) was examined 7 and 13 days after injection in each group. In every case, light led to maximal displacement, suggesting that it stimulates lamellar formation (Fig. 2.21a), though the effect is not cumulative: 2 h of light sufficed to cause 44 per cent of the observed shift in LL after 12 days as opposed to the 8 per cent expected on the basis of additivity. This is in qualitative agreement with Fig. 2.19. An additional observation points to light being more efficacious after a period of prolonged dark adaptation (Fig. 2.21b): during 24 h in LL after six days of DD the radio-active band advanced four times as fast as in darkness and 2.5 times as fast as in LL. Similarly, if six days DD were followed by LD = 12:12, then during the first 24 h after the dark period, the band advanced three times as fast as it does in darkness and twice as fast in LL. However, the rate slows down, and approaches that characteristic of LD = 12:12 used as a control. *Xenopus* tadpoles lay down disks at twice the rate of *Rana*, and Besharse *et al.* showed that most of the renewal took place during the first eight hours of illumination (LD = 12:12): the data are consistent with an exponential course having a half-time ∼ 5 hours.

A priori it is uncertain whether light acts both on the photo-receptor (stimulating lamellar growth and apical shedding) and on the pigment epithelial production of phagosomes. It is possible that the photo-pigment, partly photolysed by light-exposure, changes the internal environment of the outer limb

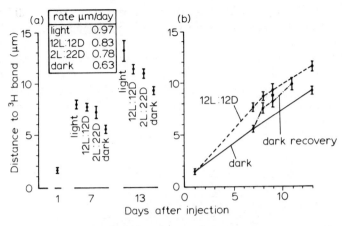

Fig 2.21 Effects of constant light, constant darkness, and cyclic light and darkness on displacement of the radioactive band in red rod outer segments of *Rana pipiens* tadpoles at 23° ± 0.5° C (cf. Fig. 2.18) (a) Distance to the radioactive band at 1, 7, and 13 days after injection in animals kept under specified conditions beginning on day 1. The inset gives the average rate of displacement in each group between days 1 and 13. Points are means of 50 to 90 measurements (ten per tadpole) from near the retinal centre except for points for constant light (means of 20 or 30 measurements). Length of vertical bars = 4σ. (b) Band displacement as a function of days after injection in animals kept on a cycle of 12 hours of light and 12 hours of darkness (12L:12D) or in darkness compared with animals exposed to the same cycle after 6 days in darkness (dark recovery). Band displacement of 2 μ during the first 24 hours of recovery corresponds to a renewal rate more than three times that in darkness. During days 2 to 4 the rate declined to one comparable to that of controls kept on a cycle of 12 hours of light and 12 hours of darkness. (From Besharse, Hollyfield and Rayborn, 1977. © 1977 by the American Association for the Advancement of Science.)

and that a rapidly moving messenger stimulates phagosomal growth. The question is amenable to experiment e.g. if one were to study a preparation with a detached or removed neural retina. It is noteworthy that rat pigment epithelium grown in tissue culture preferentially phagocytoses rod outer limbs from fully light-adapted rats. Phagocytosis of rods obtained in the dark from rats killed one hour before the onset of their accustomed light cycle is minimal. Now light exposure was not a prerequisite for this distinction: the number of outer segments increased in the dark at the time at which the light would have been turned on during the preceding photic regime. As the cultured pigment epithelium is less likely to have a memory for a cycle to which its original host is unlikely to have been subjected than is to be expected of the photo-receptors recently removed from rats subjected to a light rhythm, the notion of a messenger from apex to pigment process assumes some verisimilitude. On this view, light acts as a priming or reinforcing agent to a process that occurs at a low but non-zero level in the dark.

The discovery of circadian rhythms in the ultra-morphology of rods is able to elucidate the puzzle relating to cones mentioned on p. 85. If cones, too, have a circadian rhythm, but the work routine of different research workers studying different species respectively were also to vary, some retinal cones could appear to behave very differently from others. And this turned out to be the case.

Though similar in principle, the story happens, however, to differ in an important detail. In its final form it began to be elucidated in a study of Western fence swifts, a type of lizard (*Sceloporus occidentalis*), characterized like so many of this order by a pure-cone retina. The cones occur singly or in doublets, made up of principal and accessory cones respectively (Fig. 2.22). Prior to the examination of the retinae, the animals were kept for a fortnight on LD = 12:12 with lights on at 06.00 hours. Counts were made of phagosomes, autophagic vacuoles, and of small granules which are synthesized by the pigment epithelium.

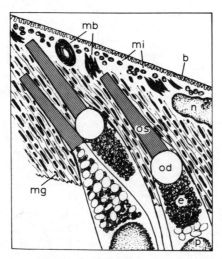

Fig. 2.22 Diagram of the pigment epithelium and the outer portions of the cone visual cells in the lizard *Sceloporus occidentalis*. mb, Circular and lens-shaped myeloid bodies in the cell body of the pigment epithelium; mi, mitochondria; b, the infolded basal surface; n, nucleus; and mg, a melanosome in one of the cytoplasmic extensions which surround the outer aspects of the cones. On the right is a single cone. os, outer segment; od, oil droplet; e, ellipsoid; p, paraboloid. In the double cone, the principal member is on the right, the accessory member on the left. (From Young, 1977. © 1977 by Academic Press Inc., New York and London.)

Fig. 2.23 shows unambiguously that phagosomes and autophagic vacuoles are approximately in antiphase with each other and that the granules obey a different circadian rhythm. That of the cone phagosomes clearly differs from that of the rods in that darkness appears to stimulate phagocytosis: it may be the case, of course, that light essentially suppresses it. Whatever the mechanism, the event takes place during the early hours of darkness.

This circadian duplicity is revealed in the mixed retina of the goldfish (*Carassius auratus L.*). Maintained for 18 days on a similar regime as the above lizards, the fish produced phagosomes which revealed two periods of activity (Fig. 2.24), one peculiar to rod ingestion in the morning, and one to cone ingestion after dark. Broadly speaking, the more highly developed retina of the chick exhibited a similarly duplex daily pattern. As before, the (male) animals had their circadian rhythm entrained during 12 days with LD = 12:12, and sacrificed on day No. 13.

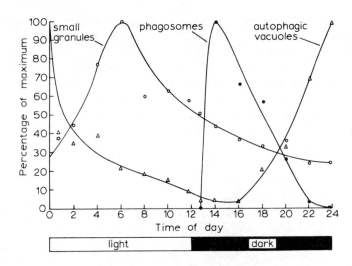

Fig. 2.23   Changes in the number of granules, phagosomes and autophagic vacuoles in pigment epithelial cells of the lizard at different times of day, expressed as a percentage of the maximum observed concentration. The time of day is given in hours, counting from the onset of the light period cf. Fig. 2.20. (From Young, 1977. © 1977 by Academic Press Inc..)

The analysis was confined to the central part of the retina, and the phagosomes were subdivided into four classes depending on the stage of degradation of photoreceptor membrane which they encompassed. Like Weale (1968) and Villermet and Weale (1969), before him, Young noted that rod and cones react differently to fixatives. Moreover, rod phagocytosis took place after the onset of light with such

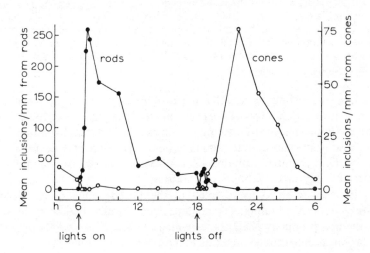

Fig. 2.24   Mean number of inclusions (phagosomes) derived from outer segment membranes at different times of day. Each point represents the mean of counts from four goldfish, including all phagosomes larger than $1\,\mu$ in the pigment epithelium and amoeboid phagocytes. Ordinates scaled cf. Figs 2.19 and 2.21. (From O'Day and Young, 1978. © 1978 The Rockefeller University Press, New York.)

speed that there was no evidence of membrane shedding after 15 minutes of light. Rods underwent photomechanical movement, heretofore observed mainly in lower vertebrates. Whereas only 25 per cent of frog rods appeared to shed their apices at any one time (p. 87), in the chick virtually 100 per cent were involved. As in the earlier studies, shedding of rod disks was intense during the first hour of the light period, and twenty minutes before its termination a few phagosomes containing cone membrane were noticed.

The cones were discarding their apices also largely within the first hours (of darkness), but the process was more diffuse than was observed for rods. Even so the rate of membrane renewal is significantly lower in cones than in rods. The latter have a turnover time of about nine days (cf. similar values for rhesus *cones*, p. 85) whereas a minimum of 23 days is estimated to hold for chick cones.

These clear results need extending to the rhesus monkey as it is unlikely that they can be confirmed directly in man. However, we are in a position to apply them to Knoerchen and Hildebrandt's (1976) study on human absolute thresholds. It will be recalled that both the cone and the rod mechanisms show a minimal threshold early in the morning (Fig. 2.17), and that the displacement of the α-point suggests different circadian rhythms for the two receptor mechanisms respectively (but see p. 80).

As yet we have no functional data with which to parallel the above ultra-morphological studies. We cannot tell, therefore, how receptor sensitivity is linked, circadially, with disk-shedding etc. It is unlikely to be out of phase with this radical event in one type of receptor, and in phase with it in the other, as Knoerchen and Hildebrandt's data might lead one to expect. There is little doubt that the no longer fashionable studies on the early receptor potential (p. 30) may provide a speedy solution to this problem.

More generally, we can now tentatively advance some ideas which may serve as budding points for discussion. The fact that rods and cones are in antiphase may help to underline some wider generalizations. The functional differences between rod- and cone-mechanisms are well-known and morphological and biophysical differences have often been noted. Although there is a well-marked difference in the electrophysiology of the two receptor types – the speed of response at threshold is greater by almost an order of magnitude in cones than it is in rods (Ch. 1) – this is unlikely to play a role under normal physiological conditions. The concept of saturation may be more useful in this connection. In general, photosensitive mechanisms respond to stimuli in a monotonic manner: the response either rises or falls. But this cannot go on forever. When a mechanism fails to increase its response even though the stimulus strength is increasing, saturation is said to occur. This is unlikely to be due to the exhaustion of unbleached visual pigment molecules. The important point to bear in mind is that, in daylight, the rods are *hors de combat* owing to saturation, but the cones do not reach the saturation stimulus level under ordinary conditions. Thus inactivity of the rods in daylight, and lack of activity of cones in the dark may respectively provide scenarios leading to the observed periodicities. Consequently, an explanation for the different circadian rhythms in the two receptor types would not be hard to produce.

It is also fairly clear that, neurophysiologically speaking, entrainment is possible at a relatively primitive level. Given a few days' training, both photo-receptors and neurones can remember when, as it were, to recharge their batteries. This plasticity and memory are key ingredients in the successful integumental layers of the animal body. The fact that entrainment can take place in the intact vertebrate eye, the crystalline lens of which transmits very little short wavelengths radiation (Fig. 1.5) does not make ultra-violet light a strong candidate for purposes of entrainment. Ordinary 'visible' light, absorbed by the rods and cones, is probably responsible, but here again simple experiments with suitable filters will quickly produce an answer.

The function of circadianism is as yet unclear, but may be a matter of bio-economics. There is no need, from the point of view of survival, to keep all functions at full tilt throughout a whole day. There is equally no reason why all the functions should go to sleep together. Once the pattern of circadian rhythms is mapped for the whole of the body, with their respective causes and effects, reasons may emerge. And with them, in all probability, there will arrive an understanding of some diseases which, at present, remain beyond it.

Questions

1 Discuss possible evolutionary advantages of circadian rhythms with special reference to an animal's metabolism.

2 Compare circadian rhythms governed by light and temperature respectively. Speculate on the role they may have played in our emergence from the sea.

3 You are asked to determine how the human visual threshold varies from hour to hour over 24-hour periods. Describe the procedure you would adopt, what precautions you would take, and what conclusions you would legitimately base on the results.

4 A coelacanth has been caught and the fishermen guarantee that it has at least 72 hours' life left. How would you set about determining whether it has a photically determined circadian rhythm?

3 Development and Age

Helmholtz, the great German physiologist and physicist, hinted that, had he been the Almighty, he would have made a better job of designing the eye than has, in fact, been the case. While the Almighty can, no doubt, look after Himself, it is only proper to stress that Helmholtz could not have known yet a great deal about the development of the eye in particular and of that of the visual system in general. The blueprint may appear to contain one or two design faults: but when one considers the overall assembly one is faced with a remarkable entity. Some features worrying Helmholtz may owe more to production than to function.

It is only during the last decade or so that the study of the development of the visual system has come to supplement the older pursuit of how the eye shapes both before and after birth. And it would be quite erroneous to dismiss this as yet another furrow to plough (or another subject to have to learn). We interact with the world and dominate it because we have learnt to handle information better than any other species. This is most valid as regards photic information. It would seem to follow that an understanding of the development of this handling ability is likely to facilitate our grasp of the working of this remarkable faculty, and that there is no need to apologize for the introduction of this topic.

However, we do not only develop but also age. Various parts of our bodies age at different rates and – horror! – do so differently in different parts of the world (Bourlière, 1970). While it would be folly to follow the sybil and to seek eternal life, there is every reason to try and extend the efficiency of all parts of the body to fit into the life-span extended now to almost a century (Comfort, 1964). This also applies to the eye. The physiology and pathology of old age are less likely to be apprehended if a knowledge of development has not first been assimilated.

We have already noted that the visual organ is part of the nervous system that depends on exteriorized tissues, and is specially adapted to absorb light (pp. 21 – 29). Embryologically the retina is derived from a germinal layer called ectoderm (which also gives rise to the lens and the skin). The photo-receptors are ciliate structures – we remind ourselves of the fortifying spine between the inner and outer limbs (Fig. 1.19) – as is true of parts of other exteriorized tissues like the respiratory tract. A brief survey of ocular embryology greatly facilitates an understanding of some anatomical functions.

When we consider the complexity of the human organ of vision we can hardly be surprised to find that its development begins within a few days of the fertilization of an ovum. A cursory glance at the earlier stages of the growth of the embryo may help to put that of the eye into proper perspective.

The two-celled fertilized ovum rapidly divides into many cells and after a short time develops into a hollow sphere (morula) which provides future housing not only for the embryo itself but also for embryonic nutrition (Fig. 3.1). An

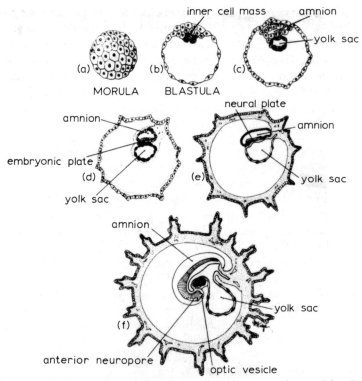

Fig. 3.1   The early stages in the development of the human embryo. (After Barber, 1955.)

accumulation of cells occurs at one pole of the sphere and represents the primordium of the developing individual. The cells of the spherical wall (blastula) have only a nutritional function.

As the sphere gains in volume, the so-called embryonal knot differentiates into two layers, namely an outer, the forerunner of the afore-mentioned ectoderm and an inner, which is made up of rapidly dividing cells. The latter line the wall of the sphere, and, after a time, give rise to another germinal layer, namely endoderm. Meanwhile, the outer layer develops the primitive streak, a structure which organizes the development of adjacent tissues. It also consists of two layers, the upper containing cells which, having passed between the ectoderm and endoderm, form the third and last germinal layer, i.e. mesoderm. The physiological differences between them have recently been found to be smaller than used to be thought in the past: the layers are even partly interchangeable. Only ectoderm and mesoderm contribute to the formation of the eye.

The next stage consists in the appearance of the so-called amniotic and archenteric cavities. The former, filled with fluid, acts as a kind of shock-absorber, the latter, provides a primitive gut which is, in fact, external to the individual. Later, there arises between them the embryonic plate in which all three germinal layers are represented (Fig. 3.1). The central portion of the plate gradually caves in to produce a groove. Its longitudinal edges rise, form neural folds and, on meeting, develop the neural tube. Because the rate of growth of the anterior end of the embryo is maximal, the plate can form a headfold: this is the name given to an upward growth of the parts which surround the anterior end of the groove. The head fold next differentiates into the three cerebral vesicles which are the precursors of the fore-brain, mid-brain, and hind-brain, respectively. The eyes are derived from the part of the ectoderm which goes to produce the fore-brain.

The first phase is completed when the optic pits are formed just after the embryonic plate has changed into the neural groove but before it has closed to a tube (Fig. 3.2a). The anterior part of the primitive brain connects the two ocular

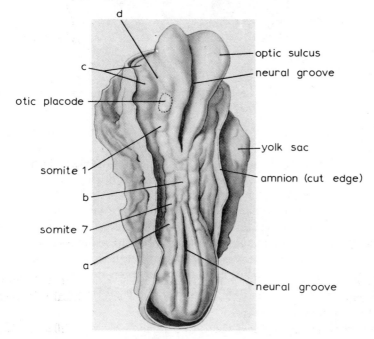

Fig. 3.2a Dorsal view of a model of a human embryo about 22 days old. (After Hamilton, Boyd and Mossman, 1945.)

primordia by means of a bridge (Fig. 3.2b) which, at an embryonic age of two months, represents the optic chiasma, where the two visual paths meet, intersect, and divide (cf. p. 39). The cells in the floor of the pit later differentiate into the rods and cones of the mature retina; i.e. the place of light absorption which initiates the visual act faces the light in the primordial eye. But because of the invagination which the latter undergoes, as will appear forthwith, nervous elements intervene between the receptors and the incident light as the eye matures (Fig. 3.3) and the retina is said to be inverted. Once the neural tube is formed the optic pits deepen and rapidly change into separate structures, the primary optic vesicles, which are each linked to the fore-brain vesicle by means of an optic stalk (Fig. 3.3a). As each vesicle grows (largely away from the fore-brain), it pushes the surrounding head-mesoderm aside until it touches the surface ectoderm.

With contiguity established, surface ectoderm begins to thicken (Fig. 3.3c), until differentiation allows one to identify lens ectoderm and later the lens plate.

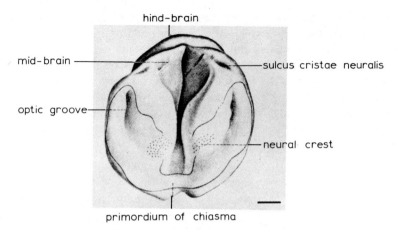

hind-brain

mid-brain

optic groove

sulcus cristae neuralis

neural crest

primordium of chiasma

Fig 3.2b   Frontal view of a model of the anterior part of a human embryo, a few days old. Bar = 0.1 mm. (After Wolff, 1948.)

Previously convex, the latter becomes slightly concave and reveals the formation of the lens pit. The changes in the surface ectoderm so far described are not specific to the cells in which they occur, but point to the existence of an 'organizer' in the pole of the primary optic vesicle. If, for instance, other surface ectoderm is juxtaposed to the vesicles or the presumptive vesicle tissue is transplanted to other surface ectoderm the same characteristic cell thickening will occur. In spite of a great deal of research having been done on them, the precise nature of 'organizers' is still undetermined, though nucleo-proteins appear to be involved. But enough is known to suggest that (a) there is more than one of them, and (b) that they can severally induce the formation of more than one organ, depending on where in the embryo they occur: their organ-specificity is said to be limited.

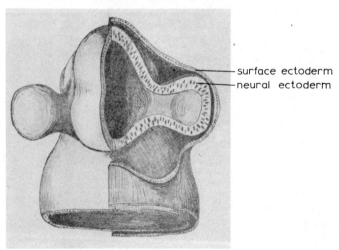

surface ectoderm
neural ectoderm

Fig. 3.3a   Model of fore-brain and optic vesicles of a ~ 20 days old human embyro seen from the front. The optic vesicle on the left of the embryo is represented in section. Note thickening of former to form lens plate. (From Mann, 1928. © Cambridge University Press.)

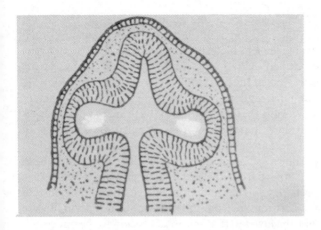

Fig. 3.3b Section of Fig. 3.3a (After Heisler, 1907.)

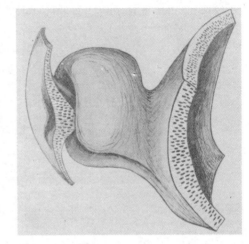

Fig. 3.3c Model of the optic cup and lens thickening of a 22 days old human embryo showing invagination of the optic vesicle to form the optic cup, and the deepening of the lens pit. (From Mann, 1928. © Cambridge University Press.)

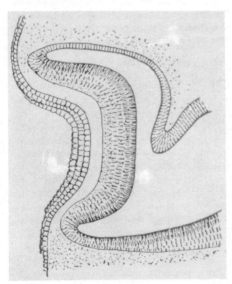

Fig. 3.3d Section of the left part of Fig. 3.3c (above) (After Heisler, 1907.)

The deformation of the lens plate leads to a series of events in the almost hemispherical shape of the vesicle. Its upper portion grows faster than any other; the lower and outer part, facing the lens plate, flattens and thickens. Its cell nuclei proliferate and – it will be recalled that we are dealing with what used to be the floor of the optic pits – form layers of the presumptive retina. The rest of the wall, however, remains one cell thick and is going to form the retinal pigment epithelium. The embryo now awaits the invagination of the primary optic vesicles.

There is good evidence to show that the power of invagination is inherent in each vesicle, and not due to mechanical pressure exerted by the thickening lens plate, although the importance of mechanical forces has sometimes been underestimated in the past. Apart from the fact that a primary optic vesicle invaginates even in the absence of surface ectoderm, invagination occurs also in the undisturbed vesicle in a part remote from the lentigenous ectoderm. Before the embryo is four weeks old, the lower part of the optic vesicle and the optic stalk begin to invaginate, forming a groove and finally the foetal ocular cleft (Fig. 3.4).

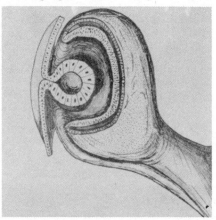

Fig. 3.4 Model of the optic cup of 4 weeks old human embryo. The wall of the cup has been cut away to show the two layers. The lens vesicle has been opened to show the cavity and the narrow passage running from this through the lens stalk. Note foetal cleft running along the bottom of the cup and stalk. (After Mann 1928.)

The latter engulfs embryonal connective tissue which contains the hyaloid artery; this is a purely foetal structure supplying blood to vessels which surround the lens (see below). The *raison d'être* of the cleft is as follows. The inner wall of the double-walled optic cup (Figs 3.3d and 3.4) is the forerunner of the retina, the outer one becomes pigmented and turns into the pigment epithelium. If it were not for the presence of the cleft (Fig. 3.4) the only connection between the presumptive retina and the fore-brain would be across the rim of the cup, i.e. through the pupil. As it is, contact between the future retina and brain is as if via a pigtail, and maintained across a short route encased in the cleft which later becomes the optic nerve. The blood supply to internal structures, such as the embryonic lens, and later, to the retina and iris is shortened by the existence of the foetal cleft.

On account of the invagination of the optic vesicle the thickening indented lens plate meets with no resistance and can, therefore, advance into the free space so provided. During the third or fourth week of the embryo's life, a lens vesicle is formed, and, at an embryonic age of about 30 days, it develops into a sphere (Fig. 3.5) which separates from the closing surface ectoderm. At this time also, the primary cells of the posterior wall elongate and fill the cavity of the lental sphere: these cells are the precursors of secondary lens fibres. Further cellular growth leads to a considerable enlargement of the lens which at one time virtually fills the optic cup. This represents an example of a general developmental principle: ontogeny (the formation of the individual) repeats phylogeny (the evolution of the race). Spherical lenses are typical of once aquatic species such as lizards and birds, and also of fish, because, in water, the cornea can barely refract, and a reinforced lens is therefore called into play.

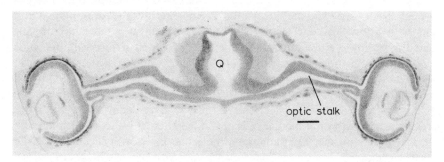

Fig. 3.5 Section through the eyes and optic stalks of a 1 month old human embryo. The fore-brain is shown at Q. The lenses are formed. Bar = 0.2 mm (After Bach and Seefelder, 1914.)

The details of lenticular development are not without interest. By about eight weeks the nuclei of the primary cells are found to have concentrated in the equatorial region of the embryonic lens. The secondary fibres arise from mitotic divisions of these nuclei and form a shell surrounding their primary precursors. The inner embryonic nucleus (easily visible with the slit-lamp in the adult eye) is lenticular and forms the centre of the lens. Fibres of the same age will be of equal length, but, as new shells come to overlie older fibres, more recent fibres are of course longer than older ones. Their lengths are, however, insufficient for them to terminate on the anterior and posterior poles of the lens, and consequently three sutures are formed. They form a Y on one side of the lens and an inverted one (λ) on the other. The advantage of sutures is evident when we consider the outer coat of a soccer ball: they bestow strength on the tissue consisting of material essentially elastic in nature (cf. Ch. 1), and, by eliminating knots from the optic axis of the eye, preserve the high optical quality of the eye as a whole. It is due to the sutures that we see stars fanning out into six streaks. (It is interesting to note, however, that the ceilings of Egyptian tombs are painted with five-streaked ones.)

From the point of view of the mechanism of accommodation it is also clear that fibres, joined along straight-lined sutures, will give rise to less overall buckling when the shape of the lens is altered than would be possible if they were knotted together at the poles.

In post-natal growth other shells are overlaid on the embryonic structure, and in frontal view obscure the appearance of the Y's. The lens continues to grow probably throughout life (p. 132).

We have seen that the retina is derived from the floor of the optic pit: its antecedent is neural ectoderm as distinct from that of the lens which is superficial ectoderm. Initially, the retinal primordium develops layers of like cells. They divide in such a way that the older cells come to lie nearer to the future vitreous: the layer of rods and cones is formed last. No further development of the retina takes place until in the sixth or seventh week when the embryo is 17 mm long. Large ganglion cells, amacrine cells, and Müller (supporting) fibre cells, are derived from the innermost cells of the nuclear zone: it is the cells of the macular region – the future region of best resolution – which develop first. The connecting fibres of the ganglion cells or axons grow along the shortest route following the shape of the optic cup through the optic stalk to the brain: the optic nerve is formed. What used to be the ridge in the foremost part of the fore-brain linking the original optic pits, now supports the optic chiasma (p. 39), produced by the partial decussation of the optic nerve fibres. At a later date (80 days), the outer cells of the nuclear zone give rise to bipolar and horizontal cells, and to the nuclei of the rods and cones.

In addition to axons, the ganglion cells develop dendrites, which give rise to the inner plexiform or molecular layer (p. 35 *seq*). The dendrites of the inner horizontal, amacrine and bipolar cells are added later (third to seventh month). The separation of the nuclear and outer molecular layers also occurs first in the macular region.

We possess more details of the development of the cat retina than that of man. Cat synapses, i.e. the gaps between efferent and afferent parts of cells, are formed before receptors. This is contrary to what is true in man; for the cat, initially blind, birth is visually a non-event. We may note in passing that, for mammals in general, birth forms a less sharp discontinuity in existence than is true of death.

Both types of receptor develop along similar lines. The original cone cells appear in the central region during the ninth week probably after development from cilia-like processes. They are each linked to the pigment layer by means of a very fine filament, the forerunner of the outer limb or cone proper. Growth continues slowly until, in the eighth month, these cells approximate to their fully developed shape. There is as yet no evidence on the stage at which the outer limbs come to contain light-sensitive material. In the rat, the appearance of detectable amounts of rhodopsin has been found to coincide with the completion of the formation of rods, although in the cat outer limb segments appear five days after birth, the pigment bearing disks being the last feature to develop. As the animal is blind at birth this observation cannot provide a paradigm for man, but is a pointer all the same: pigment is available when needed.

Very early on, the human retinal centre is more differentiated than the rest (see above). In approximately the fifth month the ganglion layer thickens in the central region, the presumptive macula (Fig. 3.6). In the seventh month the central region becomes indented (Fig. 3.7), which is why it is called the fovea. Significantly, the ganglion cell layer thins, its cells being pushed tangentially outward. The depression occurring during the seventh month is broadened to a bowl four weeks later. So that light may directly reach the cones, the ganglion cells migrate and form a layer only two deep. The bipolar layer likewise shows signs of thinning. Blood vessels fail to form in this region, which also serves to help acute vision (p. 38). When the fovea first appears the development of the

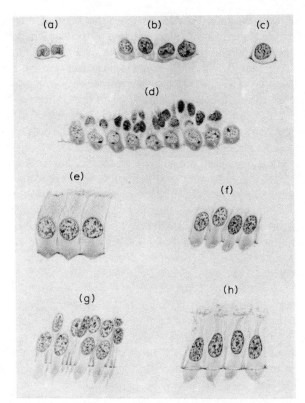

Fig. 3.6 Stages in the development of the retinal receptors. Bar $= 12\,\mu$ approx. (a,b,c) Cone cells from the central area at 9 weeks. (d) Cone cells from the central area at 13 weeks. (e) Cone cells from the central area at 8 months. (f) Cones from para-central area at 8 months. (g) Rods and cones from the para-central area at 8 months. (h) Central cones before birth. (After Bach and Seefelder, 1914.)

central area begins to lag behind that of the extramacular region, and at birth the cones are rather plump and the fovea itself does not assume its adult form until several months later. Immature as the central portion is, fixation would be very difficult even if the new-born baby had learnt to co-ordinate eye movements: the incompleteness of the foveal development at this stage may well provide a peripheral as distinct from a central cause for the baby's transitory but typical 'squint'. Accurate co-ordination between the movements of the two eyes can be of value only if the form sense is acute in each eye, i.e. if it has learnt to process high spatial frequencies (p. 14).

The cornea

Once the lens vesicle is formed (p. 98), the protoplasmic threads linking neural and surface ectoderm are invaded by mesodermal cells and we can speak of a rudimentary cornea (Fig. 3.8) in a 43 days old embryo. Throughout its development the centre of the cornea forms the thinnest part. In a sense the cornea can be considered to offer an example of arrested embryonic development: it is the only external part of the embryo to remain transparent, though at an earlier stage this is true of the whole of the embryo.

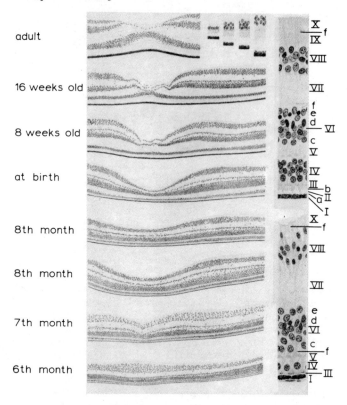

Fig. 3.7 Development of the retinal centre from the sixth month to the adult stage. I, pigment epithelium; II, layer of rod and cone (a) outer and (b) inner limbs; III, external limiting membrane; IV, layer of cone nuclei; V, outer plexiform layer; (f) Müller's fibres; (c) outer horizontal cells; VI, bipolar cells;,(d) nuclei of Müller's fibres; (e) inner horizontal cells; VII, inner plexiform layer; VIII, ganglion cells; X, optic nerve fibres. (After Bach and Seefelder, 1914.)

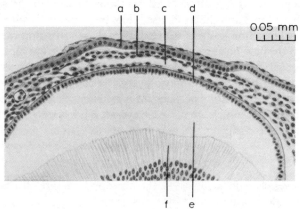

Fig. 3.8 The formation of the anterior chamber in a 6 weeks old human embryo. (a) surface ectoderm; (b) layer of mesoderm representing the future cornea; (c) narrow interval, the first sign of the anterior chamber; (d) the epithelium of the anterior surface of the lens vesicle covered by a single layer of mesodermal cells; (e) cavity of lens vesicle; (f) anterior ends of the early lens fibres. (From Mann, 1928. © Cambridge University Press.)

The sclera

Like the cornea, the sclera is mesodermal in origin. Mesoderm collects near the rim of the optic cup which, in the eighth week, reaches only to the equator of the lens. At this time there appears an opaque band of cells. Outside it, in the region of the corneo-scleral junction or limbus, there can be seen a mass of cellular connective tissue from which are derived the white sclera, episclera, and the pink conjunctiva. Inside the band, on the other hand, there forms the primordium of the ciliary muscle (p. 17). The sclera continues developing for nearly three months, the anterior being well ahead of the posterior half. This is necessitated by the development of the extra-ocular musculature.

The anterior chamber

This develops rather late in foetal life, beginning as a narrow gap in the mesoderm which is located between the cornea and the iris (Figs 3.8, 3.9). The volume of the chamber develops only after birth, partly as a result of the gradual flattening of the lens. The part later occupied by the angle (between the cornea and the external portion of the iris) is initially full of mesodermal débris. The canal of Schlemm which, in primates, drains the anterior chamber of aqueous humour, appears in the corneo-sclera during the third and fourth month, but reaches its ultimate position only during the seventh month.

The vascular tunic

The uveal tract or vascular tunic is the name given collectively to three parts of the eye: the choroid, which lines the interior of most of the eyeball, the ciliary body, and the iris (cf. Ch. 1). They form a continuous structure, and are derived partly from mesoderm and partly from neural ectoderm. Just as the primary optic vesicle acts as an organizer in eliciting the formation of the lens plate from surface ectoderm, so does the outer wall of the optic cup, the pigment epithelium, cause the surrounding mesoderm to develop the above structures.

During the seventh week the antecedents of the iris begin to form: the ectodermal tissue finding ready in position its mesodermal partner, from which the iris stroma and its blood vessels are going to be formed. Ectoderm, which provides the important sphincter and dilator musculature, lies in the rim of the optic cup (Fig. 3.9). Sphincter development begins at about the fourth month. A few weeks later this circular muscle separates from its parent cells, moves into the mesodermal portion of the iris and is invaded by blood vessels. The pupil dilator develops long after its opponent muscle has become identifiable, a circumstance that has not received any attention and may bear on a characteristic of old age (p. 132). As the radial development of the iris lags behind that of the eye as a whole the pupil goes on widening till the seventh month.

The later completion of development of the antecedent of the iridal sphincter inevitably leads to the pupil narrowing. As is well known, if it does so at all, its stroma (or basic tissue) proper does not fully develop its pigmentation until several years after birth.

Unlike the two other intra-ocular muscles, the ciliary muscle is mesodermal in origin. Mesoderm condenses during the tenth week to form the ciliary muscle.

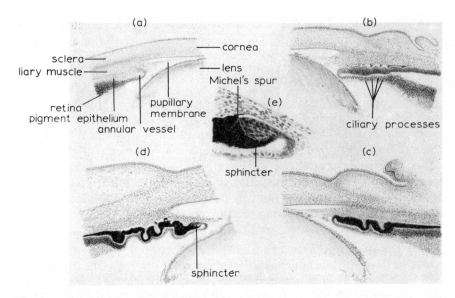

Fig. 3.9 Development of iris and ciliary body during the third and fourth months. The anterior rim of the optic cup has grown forward, and forms the epithelium of the iris, and as it does so the vessels of the lateral portion of the tunica vasculosa lentis bend round the rim of the cup (not shown). (a) anterior part of the eye of a 3 months old embryo; (b) ditto, a week later; (c) ditto for approx. 4 months; (d) ditto in the fifth month; (e) the same as (d) but under a higher power. (After Bach and Seefelder, 1914.)

Muscle fibres begin to appear at three months in a triangular area butting on, and protruding beyond, the outside of the optic cup. At five months, the meridional part of the muscle is clearly differentiated; its circular portion follows two or three weeks later.

The third member of the uveal tract, the choroid, which lies behind the retina which it provides with metabolites is a rather early part of the developing eye because it envelops the optic cup.

The vitreous body

Its origin is obscure in virtue of the fact that its development is divisible into three stages each of which produces a vitreous of its own. The tertiary, final vitreous originates in the third month when the ectodermal parts of the iris and ciliary body secrete vitreous filaments. Some of these form the vitreous and others, perpendicular to them, the suspensory ligaments of the lens (pp. 16–17).

The hyaloid and related systems

In the young embryo the optic nerve and the retina are avascular, the growing lens and vitreous being supplied by the hyaloid artery (which passes through the optic stalk) and its branching or anastomizing system. After some eleven weeks a plexus or network of veins develops round the hyaloid artery and later gives rise to two large vessels. These fuse near the optic disc, where the nerve enters the eye, and form the central retinal vein. The corresponding arteries develop a little later. These major vessels can easily be seen when one looks at night into the eyes of a cat, and form clear land-marks in the mature fundus oculi. Up to about the eighth month both the arterial and venous retinal systems continue to ramify and grow throughout the retina up to the ora serrata, the region where the ciliary body is attached to the retina. Only the veins give rise to capillaries, the arteries, or the oxygen in the blood they carry exerting some inhibiting effect. The part of the hyaloid artery running through what has now become the optic nerve is converted into the central artery. The original foetal artery supplies a system which envelops the lens. Both the artery and the vascular system atrophy before birth, but under suitable conditions of illumination, a relic – the hyaloid canal – is visible as a spiral contortion in the vitreous of the adult eye.

The extrinsic muscles

The external ocular muscles which control the position of the eye in relation to the orbit are traceable to a structure which appears during the third week of embryonic life. This is an undifferentiated massed condensation in the paraxial mesoderm which surrounds the optic vesicle. The four recti and two oblique muscles can be distinguished some four weeks later; not long afterwards the levator palpebrae superioris, the contraction of which muscle raises the upper lid, and the superior rectus, which raises the eye in upward gaze, start their development. The oculo-motor nerves are said to be observable during the fifth week, and by the end of the eighth week, they all are said to be connected to their respective muscles.

The eye after birth

When the eye at last sees light its development is still incomplete. There is evidence that some of its functions, e.g. daylight vision, cannot be fully developed without the eye being adequately exposed to light. However, the problem of what light does for the development of the visual apparatus is still controversial (Hirsch and Leventhal, 1978). This is partly due to the fact that it is plainly impossible to do experiments on human babies, and difficult to extrapolate from the development of lower mammals that may either be born blind, as happens with kittens, or be exceedingly sensitive to amounts of light thought to be harmless to man, as is true of rats. We also have to remember that, in the adult, the morphology of the visual system reveals clear circadian rhythms (p. 77): it is, of course, as yet unknown whether these exist *in utero* or, as is more likely, have to be entrained by light (Ch. 2). This may or may not be accomplished as it were overnight. But it is clear that the unravelling of the respective influences of light, circadianisms and early development is difficult even in species with which one can take experimental liberties to a degree to which this can never be true of man.

Developmental milestones

The complexity of this greatly involved situation is increased by the existence of so-called critical periods. Let us assume e.g. that the binocular interaction of the two eyes of a cat can be modified by occluding one of them. This exercise may turn out to be nugatory unless the occlusion occurs for about four weeks between eye-opening and some four months of age. There is consequently a critical period during which interaction can be interfered with: outside it, it is more, or wholly, resistant to external interference. It turns out, as we shall see, that more than one visual faculty is highly plastic during early development (Daw *et al.*, 1978), and that the critical periods do not necessarily coincide even though they may characterize cortical function.

It is hard to see why vision should be something special in this connection. It has been shown that individuals interact on a social level in a manner that appears to depend *inter alia* on whether or not they received adequate verbal stimulation and attention during infancy. Probably, this, too, requires application during some critical period. A failure to realize this may lead to a stronger though avoidable entrenchment e.g. of class distinction, and, on a more immediate level, a rich visual environment in early life is likely to be essential for the maturation of an individual's visual potential.

For this and other reasons, there has been a great deal of pressure for the earliest possible determination of infant refraction. This is not surprising. A specific stimulus is less likely to be identified if it is inadequately imaged on the retina: since the informational content of high spatial frequencies (p. 50) is considerable, a study of early modulation transfer is of great interest.

As regards its anatomy and structure, we have to remember that the infant eye is not a smaller version of its adult counterpart. This probably happens only several years after birth.

The volume of the eye-ball has yet to increase over threefold to reach maturity (the brain increases nearly fourfold, and the body as a whole over twentyfold). The shape of the eye-ball is less symmetrical than in the adult. The cornea is relatively large and, in contrast to the adult one, more curved at the periphery than the centre. The paucity of lens fibres in the neo-natal eye, and the relatively small diameter of the ciliary body cause the new-born lens to be very much more rotund than is true of the adult. This factor partly counteracts the diminished refraction of a relatively flat cornea and the hypermetropia associated with small eyeballs: as babies have more use for near than for distant vision a functional virtue is made out of a developmental necessity. The eyes gradually move further apart and tend to diverge. Although their distance apart grows with the head, ocular development may be said to be complete when the child is five or six years old.

Refraction in infants

The above-mentioned infantile hypermetropia has been known for a long time from measurements on isolated cases. More recently, records have been obtained on early variations also in astigmatism. This defect, usually associated with a slight deformation of the cornea, generally produces elongated images of small round objects. The reason is that, whereas the ideal cornea is part of a spherical surface, an astigmatic one represents optically a mixture between a cylinder and a sphere. It has consequently two focal planes with an elongated 'image' being produced orthogonally in each. Astigmatism is described as being with or against the rule, depending on whether the axis of the cylinder is horizontal or vertical. Fischer (1948) showed that the former vastly predominates in infants, and the latter in old age. However, even in early life there are marked systematic changes manifesting as a reduction of astigmatism (Fig. 3.10), and, though recent work stresses that oblique astigmatism occurs in only one out of three infants, Fischer's generalization which covered broad age-groups awaits confirmation. Howland *et al.* (1978) used a photographic technique which involves essentially flash-photography of the retinal image of an astigmatic source of light. This produces characteristic Christmas tree-top stars, the lengths of the arms of which provide a measure of defocus in orthogonal meridians.

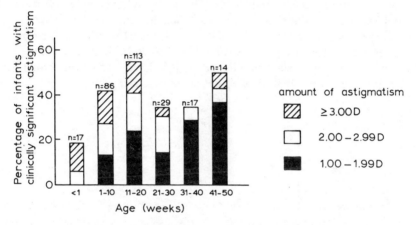

Fig. 3.10 Incidence of clinically significant astigmatism during the first year of life. The total number of infants refracted within an age group is given above each bar. (From Mohindra, Held, Gwiazda and Brill, 1978. © 1978 by the American Association for the Advancement of Science.)

The significance of these results is at least twofold. The magnitude of the astigmatic errors (~ 2 dioptres) is such as to cause telling blur at spatial frequencies resolved in the emmetropic eyes of coevals: the information conveyed by frequencies greater than about 20 c/° is therefore lost. Of greater importance from the developmental point of view is the value of high frequencies as regards the formation of the relevant cortical response mechanisms. We shall discuss below (p. 115) experiments which showed that if kittens are reared (during the relevant critical period) in an environment free from horizontal or vertical contours, orientation detectors (p. 54) for the missing directions fail to develop. The animals are said to be amblyopic for the missing direction or meridians. Such meridional amblyopia has been connected with astigmatism also in man, and the developmental significance of early undetected astigmatism was emphasized soon after the start of the current rush of studies into this important problem.

Contrast sensitivity

The above statement which suggests that, in certain meridians, the spatial frequency spectrum is much restricted (p. 15) depends to some extent on the measuring technique. As Atkinson *et al.* (1974) have shown, techniques suitable for sophisticated adults have to be modified when one is dealing with an infant less than two months old. When asked, the child will not answer and one has to have recourse to reflex movements (such as eye fixation changes) which have a much higher threshold also in adults (Fig. 3.11). It is nevertheless clear that, while the adult sensitivity is about 80 times greater than that of the infant, the cut-off frequencies (spatial frequencies for which contrast equals 100 per cent) differ by less than an order of magnitude. Note that the two sets of sensitivity curves – one obtained with flashing, the other with drifting gratings – show marked intra-set differences, but, even allowing for that, they indicate a relative displacement along both axes. They are nearest at low spatial frequencies, where the infant deficit is barely one order of magnitude. It is usually assumed that a defect at high spatial frequencies is due to optical causes (when the ocular media are clear), and we have noted that the neonate eye is hypermetropic. Though the above young observer had bilateral astigmatism, no attempt could be made to align the test-grating with the appropriate meridian: there is little doubt that this would have made the high-frequency descent of her curves less steep.

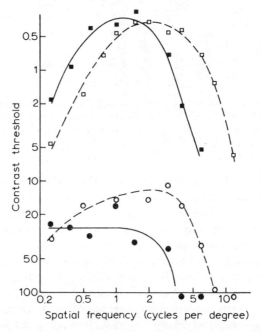

Fig. 3.11   Contrast sensitivity as a function of spatial frequency, for infant and adult observers. ■,□, Adult observer; ●,○, infant observer; ○,□, flashing gratings; ●,■, drifting gratings. Both axes are logarithmic, and the ordinate is plotted with contrast decreasing upwards. Points below the abcissa indicate values of spatial frequency for which discrimination did not reach the 70 per cent level for 100 per cent contrast. (From Atkinson, Braddick and Braddick, 1974. © 1974 Macmillan Journals, Ltd., London.)

Observations obtained with a grating drifting with 3 Hz reveal the rapidly progressive change of early development: behavioural data of the type shown in Fig. 3.12 depend on 'awareness' in a manner not so far quantified: a detailed comparison with simultaneous recordings of visually evoked responses (VER's) should be instructive in this connection (see p. 111).

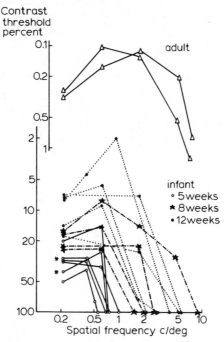

Fig. 3.12 Contrast sensitivity functions obtained for individual subjects with gratings drifting at a modulation rate of 3 Hz. The different symbols denote data from subjects in the different age groups. Note that the vertical scale for the adult data is displaced as indicated. (After Atkinson, Braddick and Moar, 1977.)

It may be noted that the meridional variations of infant visual acuity was studied recently (Gwiazda *et al.*, 1978), but the results hardly help our understanding a great deal. The tests tried to establish visual preferences of largely hypermetropic infants for vertical, horizontal, and oblique gratings of different spatial frequencies in turn. While it remains to be established that preference and sensitivity go hand in hand, oblique gratings were found to be less preferred than vertical ones. The reservation is important: the criterion of preference was deduced from the child's head and eye-movements when it was faced with two alternative test-fields. Co-ordination between stimulus orientation and movement direction also leaves it unestablished whether reaction is directly proportional to perception (cf. p. 166). It has been recently noted that the vision of (adult) cats parallels these observations. When trained to detect minimal angular differences θ with long black lines oriented on a white background along the horizontal or vertical and along oblique meridians, θ for the principal meridians ranged from 1.5–5°. For oblique ones it ranged from

~ 3–10°; i.e. the cat 'preferred' horizontal and vertical contours. This could result from astigmatism rather than neural causes.

Preferences of horizontal and vertical gratings over oblique ones were then demonstrated in infants between 3 and 11 months old. However, meridional amblyopia has not been detected before about the age of three years. Moreover, we have noted that astigmatism is systematically observed in that age-group: hence the connection between the two must be complex.

As there are several methods available for the objective measurement of infant visual acuity (which is proportional to the above-mentioned cut-off frequency), it has now been reliably shown that there is an up to forty-fold improvement in the visual resolving power of the infant eye between birth and six months of age (Dobson and Teller, 1978). There is fair agreement between results obtained with different techniques, and it is clear that 'normal' resolutions, i.e. one minute per stripe in terms of Fig. 3.13, is unlikely to be reached before an age of at least twelve months (see also Atkinson *et al.*, 1977).

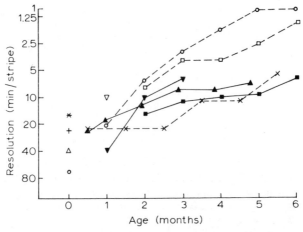

Fig 3.13 Comparison of systematic acuity data. (a) With optokinetic nystagmus (+ ×). In this technique a drum is rotated with parallel black and white stripes of variable width. If the eyes can resolve the moving grating, a reflex is set up and the eyes carry out pursuit movements. The smallest width resolved defines acuity. (b) with visually evoked potentials (▽ ○ △) (cf. Fig. 3.14 for method). (c) with behavioural tests (●▼▲ ■). (After Dobson and Teller, 1978.)

It is interesting that one of the objective techniques available for determining refraction involves not optical but electrical criteria. So-called visual evoked responses (or potentials) can be picked up with suitable electrodes placed near the 'bumps' at the rear of the head (Fig. 3.14). The wave-forms are complicated and variable, but e.g. the latent period, that is the time interval between stimulus and onset of response, offers a reliable index of the input-output situation. Now it turns out that the VER is evoked largely by cones (contrary to the electro-retinogram which is bulked from rod responses, p. 30). When the retina is stimulated with a grating then the amplitude of the VER is maximal for optimal imaging: this observation provides therefore a basis for refraction. It follows, of

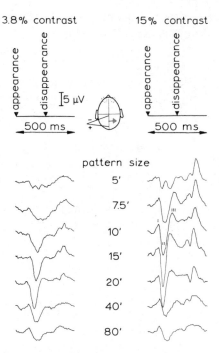

Fig. 3.14 Occipital responses to the appearance and disappearance of a checkerboard of 3.8 per cent (left) and 15 per cent (right) contrast as a function of check size. Central fixation. (From Spekreijse, Estevez and Reits, 1977. © Clarendon Press, Oxford)

course, that the VER is essentially due to high spatial frequencies (p. 14), and that the failure of the rod mechanism to respond to them explains the selectivity of the VER for cones. The infant's contrast sensitivity function (p. 109) offers poorer criteria than can be achieved electrically. Thus at three months, the cut-off frequency at approximately $4 \, \text{c}/^{\circ}$ corresponds to a little over one tenth normal adult acuity. However, the VER records at the same age (Fig. 3.13) an acuity as high as one-third normal adult (Salapatek and Banks, 1978). If this difference is significant, then it establishes that a behavioural response is less reliable than an objective one even in infants, and that the VER can throw light not only on normal but also abnormal conditions.

We are led also to some insight into the development of the infant's ability to respond, and to distinguish it from the development of its visual physiology. This distinction is not recognized by all the experts in the field. Initial short-falls in performance are not to be blamed all on underdeveloped optics or on untrained neurones. Even the retina needs at least six months of life to mature into a structure bearing comparison with that of the adult tissue. For example, in the macaque monkey whose retina resembles ours in many ways, the fovea develops continuously as regards morphology and extent from some three months *ante natum* till three or four months *post*. The central rod-free retina shrinks during three ante-natal, and ten to twelve post-natal, months to about one sixteenth of its early area: this process is accompanied by an elongation of the photo-receptor inner and outer limbs which permits progressively closer packing, and hence better resolution as the eye matures (Fig. 3.15).

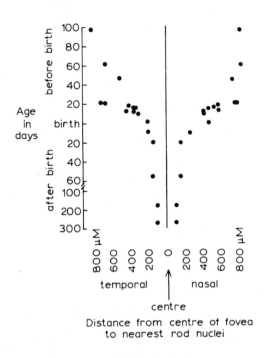

Distance from centre of fovea
to nearest rod nuclei

Fig. 3.15 Plot of the distance (in μ) from the centre of the foveal depression in *M. nemestrina* to the first group of rod nuclei. This pure cone area shows a progressive decrease in size with increasing age, with most of the decrease occurring before birth. The nearest rod nuclei are usually closer to the foveal centre on the temporal side throughout development. Some time after 8 weeks of age, the pure cone area reaches its final size of 200 μm in diameter. (From Hendrickson and Kupfer, 1976. © The C.V. Mosby Co., St. Louis.)

Fovea–stereopsis–erect posture

These details have not so far been reported for man, but probably occur also in infants. The delayed maturation of the retina provides an additional explanation for the progress in early visual development, notably that of visual resolving power and, *ipso facto*, of binocular vision. It is frequently observed that, during the first few months, infants fail to co-ordinate the movement of their two eyes: they tend to squint momentarily (p. 101). Normally, this is a reflexion of a failure in the co-ordination of the combined action of the six oculo-motor muscles, a set of each controlling the positions of the two eyes (cf. p. 105). This failure perhaps arises from an early inability to fixate which is in turn probably caused by the relatively rudimentary state of the fovea. We have to remember that the duration of human development expressed as a fraction of the total lifespan is higher than that of any of the vertebrates, a circumstance frequently attributed to man's highly evolved encephalization. At the same time, we ask ourselves whether there has been any biological pressure for the rapid development of binocular vision. In man, the perceptional fusion of the two retinal images serves one purpose: namely that of stereopsis or vision in depth.

It is arguable to what extent stereopsis is useful to an individual that spends its first weeks lying virtually immobile on its back, and at best crawls with its head up till the age of nine months. It is only when the child starts to walk that objects beyond arm's length become visually significant in the sense that it is useful to be able to gauge their spatial co-ordinates without having to touch them. At this point, then, stereopsis becomes useful. If the fovea takes six months to mature then it follows that stereopsis happens to take just as long because it needs highly developed foveal vision: the ability to resolve objects in depth is at its best for high spatial frequencies (but cf. p. 159). It is essentially at such frequencies that it is possible to divorce true stereoptic cues (such as the disparity which a given object presents to the two eyes) from other cues to depth perception such as size. The latter is clearly a low-frequency attribute, and, while aiding depth perception, does so also on a monocular basis.

It is, therefore, a remarkable coincidence – if coincidence it is – that the maturation of the fovea, stereopsis, and erect posture follow an almost causally connected temporal sequence.

To what extent retardation of foveal development is to be attributed to the highly peculiar vascular system in that area is still a mystery. The human retina is supplied by two systems (p. 2), namely the outer choroid and the inner retinal vessels. The latter are sparse in the central region, and many writers have linked this observation with the thinness of the retina in the central area. It contains virtually only cone receptors, and their metabolism, it used to be argued, could be taken care of by the diffusion gradient in the choroidal neighbourhood. The thinness of the retina is, in turn, associated with the expulsion of nuclei and neurones from the retinal centre where they might scatter light (since the retina is inverted, [p. 98]), and so interfere with the function of the area of optimum resolution. However, it has been suggested that the retina is thin because blood capillaries are absent from there. This might be due to *their* interference with vision: and the retina thins because the nuclei are expelled (or migrate) to the regions where metabolites are available, i.e. into the para-foveal regions. The older notion of an avascular central region is possibly artefactual.

However, an avascular area appears to exist in the macaque even in the foetal macula at a stage corresponding to 6–7 months' gestation in man: no report on this important question appears to exist as regards the human eye. There is clearly no visual reason for the early existence of the avascularity, and it is quite reasonable to assume that this does not exist ante-natally, as suggested by Henkind *et al.* (1975). Engerman who argues against the latter authors has shown that the macaque retinal capillary system buds centripetally, a circumstance deduced from the 'lace' appearance of the edge of the system (Fig. 3.16), but one which it is hard to understand from the point of view of actual blood-flow: why should the loops be bent rather than run straight, unless they feed into branches that have disappeared either *in vivo* or when the retina was removed from the eye? It may be argued that foveal avascularity may represent an example of arrested development. It is a matter for speculation whether this occurs because of a macular slow-down synchronizing local development with other events as

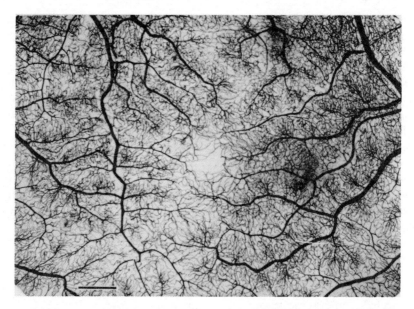

Fig. 3.16 Macular region of a normal human retina injected with Indian ink to reveal the ramifications of the retinal blood supply. Note that the centre of the fovea is not supplied by any retinal vessel. Bar = 0.5 mm. (Courtesy N.H. Ashton.)

suggested above, or whether the fovea, being a relatively late evolutionary adaptation, is trying to make up for lost time, or for some other reason.

Neuronal development

We have, as yet, no information on the detailed neuronal development of the infant retina, but, while one has to be careful in comparing one species with another and then generalizing (p. 124), we can take a brief look at what happens in the kitten. As in man, photo-receptor outer limbs of kittens are short, and the cone and rod terminals are immature and hard to distinguish from each other. This may be even more pronounced in new-born kittens, since they, unlike new-born babies, do not react to light. Their development approaches the mature state on day No. 13, but is incomplete till about week No. 5. Synapses are few and far between, and the ribbons, associated by experts in ultra-structure with active junctions near operational synapses, are also rare at three days but numerous a fortnight later. Bipolar terminals also develop their characteristic dense ground appearance only after three weeks. The cone-pedicles and their centripetal connections (p. 35) obviously mature faster than is true of the rod-system, with the bipolar layer lagging behind. But function can occur during the second week because some receptor-bipolar-ganglion paths appear to be formed. The outer plexiform layer takes some six weeks to mature. It is evident, therefore, that development appears to be patchy, and, as we shall see below, uncontrolled environmental influences have still to be considered in addition to the 'sensitive' periods previously mentioned (p. 107).

Modifying visual development

Now that we have given the peripheral, more accessible, parts of the visual path some consideration insofar as their development is concerned, we shall return to the question of how visual development can be modified by an artificial environment. For example, when kittens were raised from birth so that one eye saw only horizontal, and the other only vertical contours, their receptive fields were modified: cortical units with horizontal polar fields were obtained only for cells linked to the eye exposed to horizontal contours and an analogous situation obtained for vertical contours. Moreover, a greater proportion of these cells than usual could be stimulated only monocularly. Thus the fields only recognized contour directions to which they had learned to respond. In man, there is no need for such an artificial distortion of the retinal image to be produced in order that its potential effect on cortical development may be examined. The incidence of some sort of congenital astigmatism is relatively high: in neonates it tends to be with the rule, i.e. the axis of greater curvature is horizontal. Insofar as a strong congenital astigmatism remains uncorrected during a 'critical' period of unknown extent and position in our life-span, permanent changes in contrast sensitivity may occur. The change in shape of the function was studied by Freeman and Thibos (1975): Fig. 3.17 shows that the affected meridian exhibits a high-frequency loss. Earlier it had been demonstrated (Freeman *et al.*, 1972) that this would be due to neural and not optical factors. The cut-off frequency was measured for square and sine-gratings orientated along four meridians differing by $\pi/4$. Whereas normal observers (Fig. 3.18) had typically high cut-off frequencies for the horizontal and the vertical meridians (A), astigmats (B to E) deviated from the norm. In D and E we can see a comparison between results obtained with grating targets (dashes) and laser interference fringes (p. 13) projected on to the retina. It will be recalled that, in the latter case, the ocular dioptric system plays a secondary role: the fringes are barely affected by ametropia. The similarity between the dashed and continuous curves is evidence for the view that the anomaly lies more centrally than at the level of optics. As yet, there is no definite information on the development of the selectivity of orientation sensitive cells.

Cortical development

In kittens, striate cortical receptive fields change systematically during the first four or five weeks after the eyes open. Thus the peak value of contrast sensitivity rises by a factor of 10, a value to be compared with the results for infants mentioned on p. 109, while the acuity of the best cell rises from 0.7 to 3 c/° (Fig. 3.19). Note, however, that the cat's visual system responds in general to much lower frequencies than is true of man. There are smaller proportional changes in the response band-width (which narrows), and the best spatial frequency, which increases by a factor of 2.5 in four weeks.

It is worth noting that, at the level of the lateral geniculate body 25 per cent of the cells of normal cats show mild orientational preferences (Fig. 3.20): an arbitrary but useful criterion is provided by the length-to-width ratio of the polar diagrams. If this exceeds the value of 2, then the bias can be said to be definite. However, if kittens spend their visual life in cylinders with either horizontal or

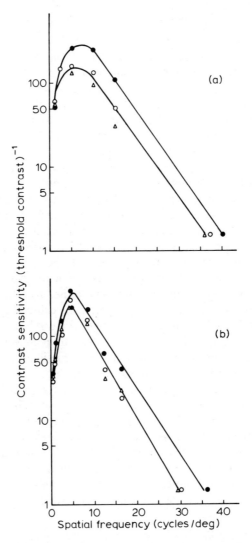

Fig. 3.17 Contrast sensitivity functions for optically corrected astigmatic observers with meridional amblyopia. The deficit is for vertical gratings, which for these observers are defocused without correcting lenses. Vertical gratings (○); horizontal gratings (●); oblique targets (△). (a) high myope with defocused horizontal lines; (b) hyperope for one meridian only. (From Freeman and Thibos, 1975. © The Physiological Society.)

vertical black and white stripes, a small relative increase in bias is observed. But the extent of the bias is affected by the rate of movement of the stimulus, if any: slow movement reveals a biased cell response but rapid movement abolishes it, as does an increase in illumination. The above and numerous other authors have shown that the orientational responses of cortical units are significantly affected by a kitten's early visual history (cf. p. 107). On reflection, the results achieved in such studies are surprising for the following reasons. Anyone who has ever

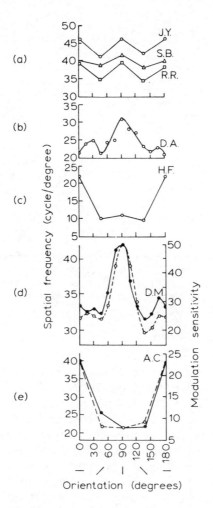

Fig. 3.18 Visual resolution of high-contrast sinusoidal or square-wave gratings that have different orientations. The ordinates on the left denote the maximum number of cycles per degree of visual angle that can just be resolved. (From Freeman, Mitchell and Millodot, 1972. © 1972 by the American Association for the Advancement of Science.)

watched young kittens must have noticed their enormous vitality. The notion that the vertical axis of their heads does not tilt is untenable: whether a set of vertical stripes is imaged more often vertically than in any other direction can only be decided by continuous cinematography and subsequent analysis of head position in relation to the environment. The presumption is made, but proof is lacking.

We stressed on p. 107 that the modification of the visual environment may interact with neural development, as just noted. But before turning to the effects of even more drastic conditions, it may be advisable to sketch a few details of what is known of the normal development of vertebrate visual pathways, notably those of the cat and monkey.

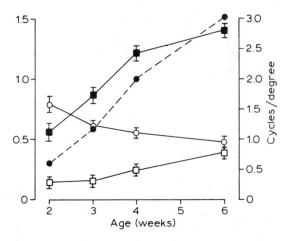

Fig. 3.19   Acuity of best cell, mean band width, mean best frequency and mean peak sensitivity for single unit recordings in striate cortex of kittens at different ages. O, band width at 0.5 height (log units, LH scale); ■, peak contrast sensitivity (log units, LH scale); □, best spatial frequency (cyc./deg. LH scale); ●, acuity of best cell (cyc/deg, RH scale). Note: contrast is defined as $(L_{max} - L_{min})/(L_{max} + L_{min})$. Contrast sensitivity is taken as the reciprocal of the contrast at threshold (L = luminance). (From Derrington, 1978. © The Physiological Society.)

One of the important developmental features relates to the differences noted for X, Y, and W-cells respectively (cf. p. 43). We recall that X-type ganglion cells have slowly conducting axons (in the optic nerve), linearly summating stimulus responses in different parts of a given receptive field, and that their response is sustained: to borrow an analogy from electricity, theirs is a d.c. response. In addition, their receptive fields are small, and the X-cells respond preferentially to low stimulus velocities. In all these respects they are distinguished from Y-cells, with rapidly conducting axons, non-linear summation, transient (a.c. type) responses, larger receptive fields; unlike X-cells, they have a low maintained discharge. The axons of W-cells are the slowest of the three, and many of the cells lack the antagonistic centre-surround (on/off or off/on) pattern associated with the receptive fields of the other two types. They appear in either tonic or phasic forms. The former show a sustained response with high maintained activity, and *vice versa* for the phasic type: consequently they represent something of a hybrid vis à vis the X and Y cells.

The above studies on lateral geniculate and cortical cells recall that the central projection of the three cell types show striking differences (Hirsch and Leventhal, 1978). X-cells lead mainly to the fore-brain: many terminate in the lateral geniculate body, and a few in the mid-brain. The LGB also receives axons of the Y-cells. But these also project on to the superior colliculus directly, and indirectly via the cortex. W-cells project also on to the superior colliculus and, less numerously, on to the cortex.

Cortical cells informed by the above cell-types reflect in their responses properties of the informants: it is as though more than one type of messenger were carried by the visual path during ontogeny. X and Y cell segregation is continued

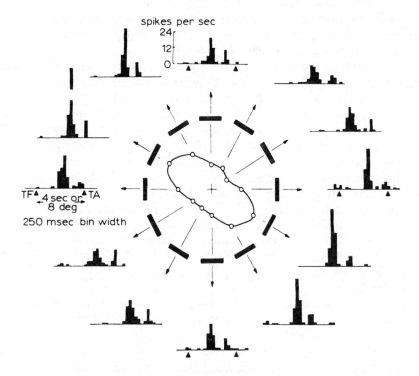

Fig. 3.20 Representative data from a computer-assisted orientation test of a cell from the cat lateral geniculate body. The cell, an off-transient unit, was tested with a black bar, swept through the RF at 2°/sec. The polar plot graphs the centre response of the unit at 12 directions of sweep. A weak bias along the 150–330° axis is apparent. The axis ratio (longest axis divided by the axis orthogonal to it) for this unit is 2.31. The data on which the polar graph is based are shown in the histograms surrounding the polar plot. A foreperiod (TF) and afterperiod (TA) are included with each histogram. Note two response peaks in each histogram, one representing a centre-and-surround response as the black bar enters the centre of the RF and leaves one side of the surround; the other, smaller peak representing the response as the black bar leaves the other side of the surround. Only the first, larger peak is graphed in the polar plot. (From Daniels, Norman and Pettigrew, 1977. © Springer-Verlag, New York.)

also at LGN level in mammals other than the cat, and, particularly in various types of monkey.

The effect of the environment would be expected to follow a hierarchical structure in the sense that a central change would presuppose a peripheral one. Nevertheless action may be indirect, as may happen when an output from the retina leads to the cortex indirectly, say, via the superior colliculi or the hypothalamus.

Hirsch and Leventhal (1978) warn against generalizations based on atypical species like rats or rabbits whose retinae show frequent signs of degeneration even in normally reared animals (cf. Weale, 1964). However, a well-controlled recent study (Chernenko and West, 1976) contradicts Rohen and Mrodzinsky's much earlier observations that the retinal layers of dark-reared animals are comparatively thin (p. 36): moreover, more synapses between amacrine and ganglion cells were observed. On the other hand, visual deprivation appears to be without effect on the development of retinal physiology.

More centrally, the situation is different. When one eye of a new-born kitten or monkey is occluded by lid suture considerable morphological changes are revealed three months later (Fig. 3.21). Those segments of the LGN that contain cells linked to the occluded eye are characterized by pyknotic changes (diminution) and cell rarefaction. However, binocular segments of the nucleus are affected more than is true of the monocular part of this relay station. Both pyknosis and atrophy may be responsible for the appearance of the areas in question, but it has also been found that dark-rearing can produce changes in response pattern from cells that show no morphological anomaly. In monkeys, pyknosis is less marked than it cats: a reversible 15 per cent reduction in perikaryal (cellular) cross-sectional area results from monocular deprivation lasting for a week or two after birth. Recovery is, however, confined to the first two months of life. It is noteworthy that binocular deprivation produces a smaller morphological effect than does monocular interference, but it is spread throughout the whole of the lateral geniculate body.

Recent work has shown that the functional division of retinal ganglion cells into X, Y and W cells (p. 43) is particularly significant in the context of visual deprivation, and, by implication, of post-natal development. The percentage frequency of Y-fields, expressed in terms of the sum of X-and Y-fields in the

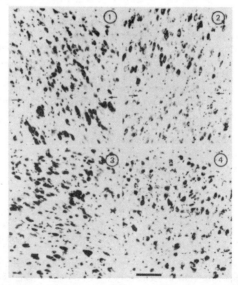

Fig. 3.21 (1) Binocular segment of laminae A and A1 from contralateral lateral geniculate nucleus. Small cells of lamina A are in upper part of figure and larger normal cells of lamina A1 in lower part. Arrows indicate interlaminar zone. (2) Binocular segment of laminae A and A1 from ipsilateral lateral geniculate nucleus. Small cells of lamina A1 are in lower part of figure and larger normal cells of lamina A are in upper part. Arrows indicate interlaminar zone. (3) and (4) Monocular segments. Note there is no significant cell shrinkage in this segment of the nucleus. Bar = 15 μ. (From Guillery and Stelzner, 1970. © Wistar Press, Philadelphia.)

normally reared cat, showed drastic drop in the binocular segment (Fig. 3.22) with projection from the occluded eye: the X-field density was unchanged but many of the receptive fields were abnormal, no matter whether lids were sutured or the animals reared in complete darkness. A reduction in the binocular inhibitory interactions between neurones of the cat's lateral geniculate body is observed following binocular deprivation suggesting that, in normal development, the neurones learn 'discipline'. If the Y-cells mediate some of these inhibitory influences, this observation would receive a simple morphological explanation.

The loss of Y-function is also reflected in the developmental physiology of the cat's superior colliculi, centres which are concerned not only with the control of eye movements but also with visual attention. While the adult colliculi therefore contain direction and motion-sensitive cells together with those that receive information from both eyes, their numbers are sparse in the eyes of the new-born: visual experience, not just growth, is vital for their full development. Graded in

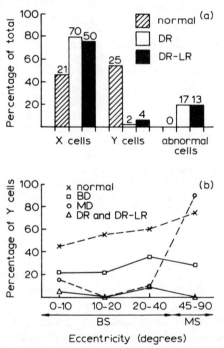

Fig. 3.22 Cell types in the dorsal lateral geniculate nucleus. (A) Percentages of X cells, Y cells, and abnormal cells in normal cats, two dark-reared cats (DR), and two dark-reared cats that received subsequent normal visual experience (DR-LR). The number of cells in each group is shown above each bar. Note both the decreased percentage of Y cells and the number of abnormal cells in animals reared in the dark compared with normal cats. (B) Comparison of percentage of Y cells in normal cats, cats in which the eyelids were binocularly sutured (BD), the laminae of deprived cats with monocularly sutured lids (MD), and the four cats reared in the dark. The data are broken down into groups on the basis of the eccentricity in the visual field of the receptive fields sampled. Abbreviations: BS, binocular segment (the central portion of visual field, imaged in both eyes); MS, monocular segment (the peripheral portion of visual field, imaged only in the ipsilateral eye). (From Kratz, Sherman and Kalil, 1979. © 1979 by the American Association for the Advancement of Science.)

accordance with their velocity response, cells responding to angular speed show that a normal environment promotes the development of high-speed detectors at the expense of low-speed ones (Fig. 3.23), again a feature that may be associated with the corresponding situation observed for the Y-cells.

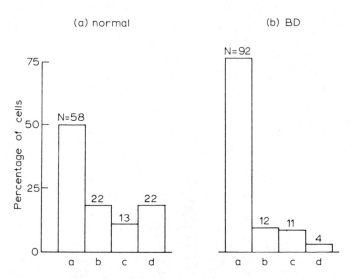

Fig. 3.23 Selectivity for speed of stimulus movement measured in superior collicular neurons of normal (left) and binocularly deprived (right) cats. For each, horizontal axis indicates preferred stimulus speed groupings as follows: a, neurons preferring speeds of less than 5°/s (in binocularly deprived cats, these cells mostly responded only to stimulus speeds less than 1°/s); b, neurons responding to speeds well over 100°/s. Vertical scale gives percentage of a, b, c, or d neurons in each group. (From Hoffmann and Sherman, 1975. The American Physiological Society, Bethesda.)

Cortex: ruler or follower?

It is a moot point whether the cortex, being more central than the above-mentioned stations, exhibits developmental anomalies much as a broad river carries the pollutants of all its individual tributaries, or whether it responds, through them, with greater sensitivity on account of its plasticity. The fact remains that the numerous factors determining the situation render adequate control correspondingly harder even though synaptogenesis starts before the animal's birth. Nevertheless synaptic connections that fix cortical performance are finalized well post-natally. For example the dendritic spines of the pyramidal cells in layer V of the mouse cortex follow a bi-modal time-course of density growth. They reach half their final value a fortnight after birth, irrespectively of the milieu wherein the animals (mice) are reared. Darkness retards development after this stage is reached. Subsequent illumination leads to normal spine numbers after another week or so. In permanent darkness, however, normality is achieved in animals twice as old as those reared in the light (Fig. 3.24).

Similar changes have been observed in other species including, e.g. in the apical shafts of the pyramidal cells in layer III (Fig. 1.37) of primates. However, density

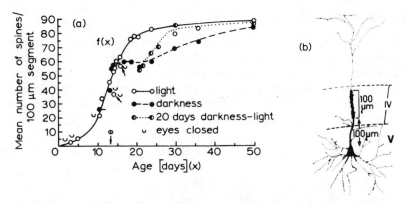

Fig. 3.24 Effect of deprivation on development of dendritic spines in visual cortex of mouse. (a) Mean number of dendritic spines per segment in apical dendrites of layer-V pyramidal cells of visual cortex as a function of age. (b) Location of standard segment in which number of spines has been counted on each apical dendrite. (From Valverde, 1971. ©Elsevier/North-Holland Biomedical Press, Amsterdam.)

estimates of the number of synapses per cortical neuron as a function of a kitten's age are hedged with difficulties associated with the accumulation of non-relevant tissue. While their number grows rapidly once the kitten opens its eyes on its eighth day (Fig. 3.25), an apparent decrease occurs at the age of five weeks. As atrophy is unlikely at this age in the normal cortex, the postulate of an increase in inter-neuronal distance (see pp. 124–127 below) seems more reasonable. Suppression of photic impulses is said to cause a reduction in the synaptic population notably of layers IV and V of the feline visual cortex. These changes appear to be irreversible.

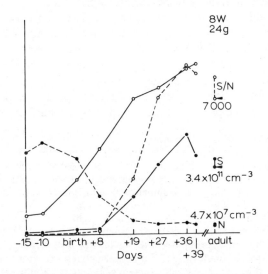

Fig. 3.25 Growth of brain weight (W), density of synapses (S), density of cell nuclei (N), and number of synapses per neurone (S/N) in 8 kittens and 2 adult cats. (From Cragg, 1972. © The C. V. Mosby Co., St. Louis.)

Species differences

In the visual cortex of squirrels, total monocular deprivation leads to a possibly compensatory increase in neuronal density in the hemisphere contralateral to the occluded eye, both in the monocular and the binocular segments. But in the cingulate part of the cortex, contrary to what is observed in the cat, there is no difference between the two hemispheres. It is noteworthy that the cortical changes resulting from light deprivation in the squirrel must be independent of those occurring in the (more peripheral) lateral geniculate body: perhaps the latter depends on differentiation between the inputs from the two eyes. We recall again (cf. p. 49) that, more than a real species difference, the difference between squirrel and cat may lie in one animal having lateral eyes and the other frontal vision. In cats and monkeys, where there is the columnar and sheet arrangement described on p. 49, early rearing determines the representation of the two eyes severally and combined. For example in monocularly deprived monkeys, the preserved system is enlarged in comparison with its area in the normal animal. This may be due to the fact that shifts in the ocular dominance of cortical neurones may be accompanied by atrophic changes.

The physiological function of the striate cortex seems to have both innate and acquired properties, although there appears to be some controversy as regards orientation-sensitive neurones, cells, it will be recalled, which are associated hypothetically with meridional astigmatism (p. 107). There is a suggestion to the effect that the orientation specificity of cortical cells responding to the stimulation of retinal X-ganglion cells (p. 43) is determined ante-natally, whereas Y-links involve visual experience. Other experiments tend to confirm a distinction between X and Y-links in the developmental context: in particular, it is the morphology of cortical cells linked to Y-cells that is likely to be affected by visual deprivation in that inhibitory responses are suppressed.

It is worth nothing that, in lateral-eyed species like the mouse, rabbit and rat, post-natal deprivation reduces the rate of, but does not vitiate, successful development. In cats and monkeys there are consequences for orientational sensitivity and also for binocular dominance (Wiesel and Hubel, 1974): the distribution depends not only on the duration of lid closure but also on the animal's age when it occurs (Fig. 3.26). In both cat and monkey, binocular deprivation reduces the proportion of binocular potentially active elements, and

Fig. 3.26 Ocular-dominance histograms for different visually deprived monkeys. (a) Monkey No. 1, binocular closure 2–17 days. (b) Monkey No. 2, binocular closure 0–30 days. (c) Monkey No. 3 binocular closure 2–38 days. (d) Monkey No. 4, normal 21-day-old-monkey. (e) Ocular-dominance histogram for area 17 in 28 normal adult (and juvenile) monkeys. (f) Monkey No. 5, binocular closure 21–49 days. Definition of ocular-dominance groups: cells of group 1 driven only by contralateral eye; for cells of group 2, marked dominance of contralateral eye; for group 3, slight dominance. For cells in group 4, no obvious difference between two eyes. In group 5, ipsilateral eye dominated slightly; in group 6, markedly, and in group 7 cells driven only by ipsilateral eye. Shaded areas at bottom of each histogram indicate period during which one eye or the other was closed. Shaded areas in histograms themselves represent cells that give abnormal responses, e.g., lack of orientation specificity or unusual sluggishness. Dotted bins to right of histograms (C) and (F) represent cells that failed to respond to either eye. (From Wiesel and Hubel, 1974. © Wistar Press, Philadelphia.)

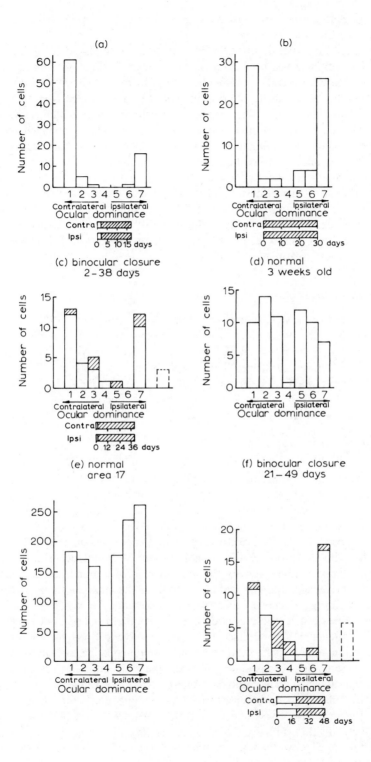

(a)

(b)

(c) binocular closure
2 – 38 days

(d) normal
3 weeks old

(e) normal
area 17

(f) binocular closure
21 – 49 days

this deficit is greatest amongst neurones with small receptive fields, i.e. those subserving the areae centrales.

Although binocular deprivation informs on the role played by light in visual development, little has been done so far as regards the determination of the relevant spatial spectral components, if any. In monocular deprivation, some attention has been paid to filtering of spatial frequencies, as is implicit in the suppression of contours. When monocular occlusion in the kitten is alternated, the number of orientation-sensitive neurones remains unchanged, but the number of cells responding to binocular stimulation drops. This occurs also in both monkey and cat, when binocular correspondence is disrupted e.g. by the severance of an extra-ocular muscle. This has a clear bearing on the relevance of early squints to cortical development. Monocular deprivation shows its effect during 8–12 weeks following the first four weeks of a kitten's life. A few hours' monocular exposure during the critical period suffices to reduce binocular interaction in kittens, a result of significance in connection with patches used clinically in the treatment of squints.

Critical periods

The plasticity of the visual cortex of kittens is asynchronous for different stimuli. For example, a preponderance of neurones responding preferentially to stimuli moving from left to right can be produced by rearing animals inside a rotating drum lined with vertical stripes. This is probably due to the absence of the reverse stimuli. The critical period for this stimulus deprivation ends after 5–6 weeks of life. Monocular deprivation, on the other hand is effective during the first 8–10 weeks: an animal reared with only, say, the left eye open will have nearly all its cortical cells driven by that eye (cf. p. 125 for the dominance pattern in normal animals). If lid-suture is reversed in time, i.e. at five weeks, more than 75 per cent of the cells will, however, be driven by the eye opened second. With an analogous reversal in drum rotation the 'reverse preference' cells will double in number. In general, stimulus change of two types leads to a summation of effects perhaps because a given cell responds to both directional sensitivity and binocularity (Daw *et al.* 1978), but the fractional changes effected at one point in time are dissimilar because the relevant critical periods do not coincide. It is not surprising that the critical period for directional responses should occur early in life. Learning co-ordination between the movement of the retinal image and body movement depends on them, and is essential for the animal's stability. It is less necessary for aggressive activity than is true of binocular vision (cf. p. 49).

The delineation of these periods is not abrupt. In a brief but penetrating survey, Mitchell (1979) stresses that the sensitive periods for orientational modification and for meridional amblyopia do not coincide, and below we draw attention to complications arising for example from problems associated with refraction, and partial accommodation (p. 129): Van Sluyters reared kittens normally for 32 days, and then deprived them monocularly for 10 days. At this point, the sutured eye was opened and the open eye closed. We may mention parenthetically that suturing is very much less effective than dark rearing, and is probably less effective than an opaque contact lens, which may, however, entail problems for the ocular exterior.

Following periods of reverse suturing which lasted from 6 to 14 days recordings were made from cortical cells so that their population might be established. The variation in the ocular dominance pattern demonstrates how they change (Fig. 3.27). (a) indicates the control stimulation with the deprived right eye remaining closed: the left dominates the response pattern. A fortnight's subsequent exposure of the right eye, the left having been sutured instead, has led to an almost complete reversal with only some neurones not sensitive to orientation preserving their original dominance (or developing it during that time interval). The hypothesis advanced on the basis of these studies is that short-term deprivation leads to reversible silencing of synapses remaining otherwise intact, whereas prolonged interference with the normal stimulus pattern causes disruption of the relevant pathways (cf. p. 128). We have noted the differential effects associated with X- and Y-paths, and may note also that studies with evoked potentials confirm the view that fast afferent paths reveal after deprivation a greater reduction in activity than is true of slowly conducting

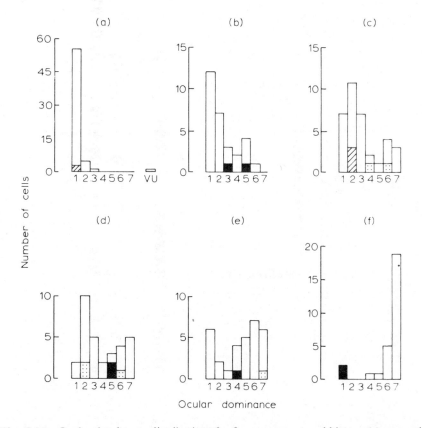

Fig. 3.27 Ocular dominance distributions for five reverse-sutured kittens. (a) comparison data from three kittens monocularly deprived from day 32 to day 42 and not reverse sutured; (b) histogram for a kitten deprived from day 32 to day 42 and allowed 6 days of deprivation reversal (d.r.); (c) 8 days of d.r.; (d) 10 days of d.r.; (e) 12 days of d.r.; (f) 14 days of d.r. Receptive field types: orientation selective = unfilled; orientational bias = stippled; pure direction selective = diagonally striped; non-oriented = filled; visually unresponsive = VU. (From Van Sluyters, 1978. © The Physiological Society.)

paths. Evoked potentials might provide a useful non-invasive monitoring technique but it cannot as yet give the detail illustrated above.

At the cortical level functional reversal occurs both in kittens and in baby monkeys, and is well-illustrated in Fig. 3.28 for cells outside layer IV$_c$ (cf. p. 47). All monkeys were initially deprived in the right eye (whence the left eye dominated). Note the similarity between this figure and Fig. 3.27. The cells were generally orientation-sensitive and after reverse suturing at 5.5 weeks became dominated almost wholly by the new visual experience. Note that intermediate reversal led to partial recovery.

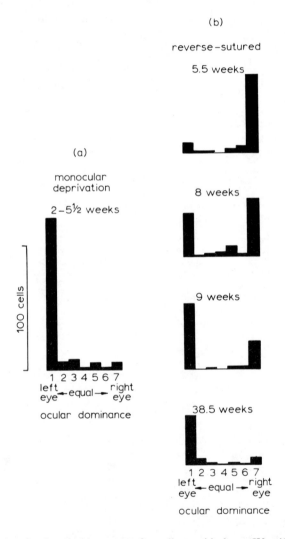

Fig. 3.28 Ocular dominance histograms for cells outside layer IVc. (Groups 1 and 7 = cells dominated monocularly by left and right eyes respectively. Group 4 = equal influence from each eye.) All monkeys initially deprived in the right eye. (a) control. (b) reverse-sutured at ages shown and left for 4 months. (From Blakemore, Garey and Vital-Durand, 1978. © The Physiological Society.)

Visual performance

With the above well-documented physiological changes occurring at relatively peripheral stages of the perceptive behavioural loop, we face the question of precisely what bearing they have on an individual's visual performance. Remember that their relations e.g. to meridional amblyopia is still a matter of surmise: no one has opened an amblyope's brain and been able to point at anomalous cells. For all that, the pointers are suggestive.

However, a series of studies has indicated that interference with the normal environment of a developing individual does lead to optico/visual impairment amenable to quantification, and, thereby, to predictions as regards behaviour. For example, it is possible to measure the spatial resolving power of an individual neurone of the lateral geniculate body by first determining its receptive field and then scanning it with high-contrast gratings of variable frequency: the maximum frequency to elicit a correlated response defines its visual acuity. In monocularly deprived kittens, Maffei and Fiorentini (1976) found that neurones of the deprived eye had, after three months' suturing, about one half the acuity of open-eye neurones. Similar results were reported on macaque monkeys. Three had one eye-lid each sutured at the age of three weeks. One of them had the central $10°$ of the visual field coagulated with an argon laser. At the age of nine months all three were reverse-sutured, and a second animal was also argon treated in the open eye. Among monkeys, as in cats, older animals can recover from monocular deprivation if the unoccluded eye is removed: even acuity improves in the previously occluded eye. The second of the above monkeys behaved normally within two weeks of suture reversal. If the open-eye retina is removed within the critical period, few of the effects of monocular deprivation can be prevented (Hendrickson *et al.* 1977). Since interrupted suturing has yielded evidence to suggest that the ocular dominance pattern (in lambs) can be changed in the course of one hour, morphological studies are still premature: but their potential relevance to the discussion on p. 126 will be obvious.

Refraction, darkness and sleep

It is also interesting to note that dark-rearing may affect the refractive state of the eyes. If lids are sutured—which can lead to lid fusion—when monkey babies are a week old, the sutured eye is found to be myopic in excess of 10 D 12 months later. This axial myopia is said to result from an elongation of the posterior segment of the eye (Wiesel and Raviola, 1977), and raises the question of whether the gradual decrease in neonatal hypermetropia as the infant gets older may not be due simply to babies doing a lot of sleeping in daylight. When monkeys are reared in the dark they develop myopia only if transferred from darkness to an illuminated habitat. However, myopia in monkeys has not been observed in all such tests, and the mere caging of the animals may play a role in this respect. Species differences may also play their usually nefarious role. Thus, when kittens were reared in the dark, except for a daily hour or two when they wore a high-power negative lens in front of one eye, their cortical units exhibited anomalous contrast sensitivity functions (p. 117) when tested with gratings of variable contrast and frequency. The ocular dominance pattern revealed a shift toward the normally focusing eye, though less so than would be obtained after monocular occlusion: cells monocularly driven by the defocused eye tended to have low cut-off frequencies (cf. p. 15).

Visual behaviour, visual functions and hazards

If, then, visual experience plays a relatively obscure, but increasingly more definite role in the development of the brain, the extent of the influence of light in the maintenance of the efficacy of the visual system is still little charted. We noted in Ch. 2 that certain circadian rhythms depend on light: in spite of sporadic reports to the effect that light deprivation, or even only that of some spectral components, can produce permanent deleterious changes, it is obvious that nothing definite has so far been established for man.

What is noxious and what unpleasant may also constitute a problem. For example, there are persistent reports suggesting that a minority of people dislike fluorescent lighting. There is no known physiological reason why this should be so. However, if they dislike it for a sufficient length of time then they may be harmed as with any other phobia. It is unlikely, however, that this harm can involve the visual, as distinct from the perceptual system of the informational loop.

Then there is the question of 'close' reading. This used to be said to harm sight and, according to a recent report on myopia suddenly appearing in a Labrador community (Johnson *et al.* 1979), this notion is still believed. It is unlikely that the mere act of seeing something close can be harmful: the visual pathway is unlikely to be anything but indifferent to the size of the retinal image. However, if there is stress this will be muscular. Close vision requires considerable accommodation and, with it, convergence of the visual axes, the two faculties being linked by a reflex, just as they are to pupillary miosis or constriction. The latter device serves to increase the depth of focus by reducing the untoward effects of spherical aberration. Children can accommodate by about 12 dioptres, that is to say they can focus an object only 8 or 9 cm away from their eyes (Fig. 3.29). It can be argued that a persistent exercise of the ciliary muscle, involved as it is in constriction during accommodation, may lead on the steady-drop principle to a permanent change in the shape of the anterior ocular segment and push it in the direction of myopia. The strong action of the extra-ocular recti muscles, needed for convergence, may similarly lead to permanent deformation. Whether all this is true is undecided; but it has been shown that myopia can be induced in monkeys kept in a visually confined space.

The evidence as regards benefits bestowed by some colours, and harm caused by others, is also largely unsubstantiated. Green used to be said 'good for the eyes'. But the reason(s) for this dogma always fell by the wayside. This did not prevent, 'black' boards and operating-theatre linen from being produced in a murky green, perhaps on the principle, in the latter instance, that it makes the patient look pink by contrast.

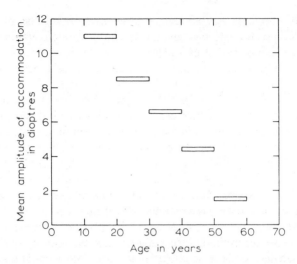

Fig. 3.29 The senile decrease in the amplitude of accommodation. (After Brückner, 1959. From Weale, 1963. © 1963 H. K. Lewis & Co. Ltd.)

Light exposure and age

Apart from self-evident mechanical hazards, the principal 'user' stimulus potentially damaging, or at least modifying, vision is without question strong light. Simple considerations of focus and radiometry make it clear that the sun can burn the retina when it is fixated for as little as two seconds or less. It is not a proposition to be verified by experiment. More insidiously, it is possible that life-long exposure to relatively high doses of ultra-violet radiation may lead to changes in the properties of the crystalline lens. For example, people living near the equator may have yellower lenses than their more Northern coevals. That this may have long-term secondary effects on vision is exemplified by the eye of the rudd.

This contains not only a colourless lens liable to turn yellow when the fish is some six years old, but also a visual pigment in its rods with a carotenoid chain that changes Summer and Winter. It can be shown that this change fails to occur after the sixth or seventh year of life: the fish is left permanently with its Winter pigment, presumably because the yellow lens mimics Winter photically. Although the human lens progressively yellows as we age, no one seems to have addressed himself specifically to the question whether this is liable to modify the photochemical constitution of the retina by modifying the photic environment wherein it finds itself.

We noted that light *qua* light has been thought of as a noxious agent (Ch. 2), and Marshall (1979) believes that the ultra-structural changes he has reported in senile retinal receptors may arise from the effects of cumulative light exposure. Without additional hypotheses, the turnover rate of some four weeks for primate cones limits the probable validity of this interesting notion (p. 91). Nevertheless, we have to face the fact that we live longer and longer: liberties which we may have taken with our bodies two centuries ago when they lasted for about half their present lives may become unacceptable if we wish to stretch their existing potential. This supposes that part of our make-up consists of capital whereon to draw, as on a depleting store of energy. We have to beware, however, lest we identify aging with depreciation, deterioration, etc, just because the outward manifestation of the underlying processes encourage mechanistic analogies. It is just as likely that we are involved in an overpowering process of forgetting – forgetting what we learnt, forgetting inborn processes, forgetting imitation, forgetting how to remember. If this leads to errors in protein replication then cumulative tissue disorganization can be envisaged without external agents.

Presbyopia

With increasing life-spans, characteristics of old age may be with us for a long time or may come to start later in the foreseeable future. In the West, the menopause starts later than it used to, and, to return to the eye, presbyopia (Fig. 3.29) starts later in the United Kingdom and Sweden than, e.g., in Cuba, India, and Somalia. As there is very little indication of assimilation occurring as between e.g. Pakistanis and the indigenous population of the United Kingdom, it will be interesting to compare the onset of presbyopia amongst the immigrants and their ethnic root country respectively.

Presbyopia is the sight of the old. Specifically, it denotes a failure of the lens to accommodate for near vision, the reason for which was thought till a decade or two ago to lie in a hardening of the lens. Remember that, no matter which modern view we adopt, all theories of human accommodation presuppose that the lens changes its shape during accommodation, i.e. that it is subject to phakomorphosis. A questionable manner of reasoning led earlier to the view that, if it cannot change its shape, it must be hard as a stone, since stones cannot change their shape either. The idea that the old lens is sclerosed (i.e. glassy) was adopted by many who had never examined normal lenses. Now it is true that young human lenses are softer than old ones: but hard normal lenses are unusual in man. To meet sclerosed lenses one has to turn to those of fish, which can barely be transsected with a scalpel, and which incidentally do not change their shape at any time: where piscine accommodation exists, it is achieved by phakokinesis, or lens movement.

Presbyopia is a multifactorial phenomenon: while permanent elastic changes in the zonule and lens matrix, changes in the stored energy and shape of the lens, modification in zonular tension, and shape alterations in the ciliary muscle all contribute to ultimate focusing failure, they occur non-uniformly and, as stressed above, with different geographic distributions, probably determined by environmental temperature.

Senile miosis

However, vision does not consist only of focusing even though, in vertebrates, an image is a *sine qua non*. For example, there occurs a subtle systematic change in its intensity. We noted (p. 6) that this is governed not only by the brightness of the objects as would be expected, but also by the area of the pupil and the transmissivities of the ocular media. The role of the pupil is significant. It grows during the first few years of life more or less in step with the growth of the ocular tissues as a whole. Unlike they, however, it reaches a maximum in the early teens. We must not allow such comparisons to confuse us: the pupil is not a tissue but a void, even though physiologically a highly functional one. After the age of 12 – 15, its diameter decreases with age (Fig. 3.30). Put another way, the iridal annulus becomes wider as we age. Does this remove an apparent paradox? Does it mean that the iris goes on growing when other tissues have stopped increasing in volume?

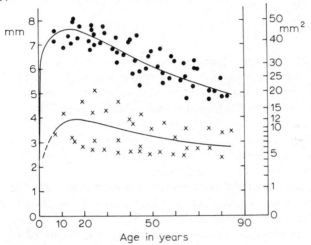

Fig. 3.30 Age variation of pupillary diameter and area. Points: dark-adapted eye; crosses: light-adapted eye. (After Verriest, 1971.)

It seems that the iris offers an example of early atrophy. It does not rigidify, as erroneous clinical opinion has been known to hold, but rather manifests the declining antagonism between the iridal dilator and sphincter respectively (Fig. 1.3). Remember that the pupillary area is determined by the tonic activity of these two muscular systems. All that needs postulating is that the two involuntary muscles share the characteristics of other smooth (unstriped) muscles, namely that they tend to atrophy with age. If the weaker of the two, i.e. the radial dilator, atrophies faster than does the sphincter, the pupil must constrict, admitting less and less light to the retina as we age. It is useful to remember that, at the age of 60, our eyes receive about one third of the quantity they used to receive at 20.

Lenticular absorption of light

But the pupil is not the only photic bottle-neck. We cannot take high transmission factors (Fig. 1.5) for granted, certainly not in the visible part of the spectrum. The light absorption of the lens, relatively high in the blue and violet parts of the spectrum even in the young, rises dramatically after the age of 40 (Fig. 3.31).This increase in optical density seems to consist of two components: on the one hand, the aging lens scatters more light, particularly the short

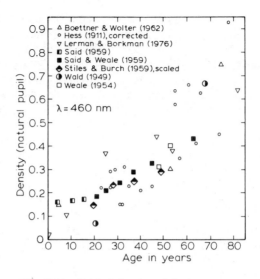

Fig. 3.31   Optical density of the lens vs age.

wavelength variety; on the other, there is a progressive accumulation of a yellowish substance. The upshot is that the lens becomes optically denser particularly at short wavelengths.

In extreme, pathological conditions, this situation is accentuated in the guise of a brunescent cataract. We obtain an idea of the filtering effect of such lenses when we remind ourselves that, on having his cataractous lenses removed, the aged French painter Monet tried to repaint some of his canvases because they appeared too blue to his eyes, freed from blue-absorbing filters.

Thresholds and visual resolution

It is found that the visual threshold (cf. p. 78) rises systematically throughout life, and much of this increase can be accounted for in terms of the above physical causes. However, in common parlance, vision is understood to mean not sensitivity (p. 28) but the ability to resolve fine detail: 'Is your vision good enough to spot the future beauty queen?' or 'Is your vision up to reading the registration number on that car?'. We saw in Ch. 1. that this aspect varies e.g. with the contrast of the target, but can be generally defined by the cut-off frequency (p. 12). This is in the region of $60 c/°$. This frequency is found to vary inversely with age, a finding only partly explicable in terms of senile miosis.

The above-mentioned increase in lenticular light-scatter can cause a deterioration of the retinal image. This provides a qualitative explanation for the loss of visual resolution, but, under normal conditions, cannot do this quantitatively on its own. A more significant factor seems to be cell-death. Various parts of the central nervous system have been shown to decay piecemeal at the rate of a few per cent per decade, and the retina forms no exception: in its later years it is found to contain progressively larger numbers of disrupted receptors (Fig. 3.32). If one assumes that cell-death occurs in a random manner, and that it does so at the same

(a)   (b)

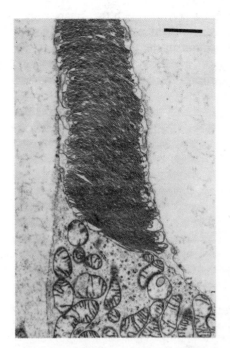 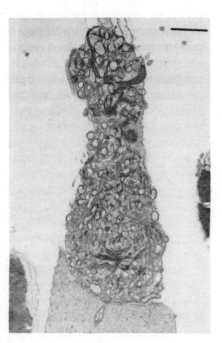

Fig. 3.32 Electron micrographs of the outer segments of cone cells in (a) 28-year-old, (b) 75-year-old, person. The vesicular degeneration in (b) is associated with the normal aging process, but may also be related to the light history of an individual eye. Bar $= 1\,\mu$. (From Marshall, 1978. © Excerpta Medica.)

rate e.g. in the receptor layer as in the lateral geniculate body, it turns out that only some half a dozen such stations need to be postulated to exist between where light acts and where the decision is made that resolution has occurred. This is not an expected result: wherever one may believe that consciousness resides one would not expect it to stick its neck out as peripherally as all that. Yet the notion that the visual cortex – only some four stages away from the outside world – should partly house our visually evoked decision-making processes is not unattractive. It remains to be seen whether this opinion is based on more than a deduction resting fortuitously on the simple fitting of a logarithmic function.

On a more general note, the study of aging of the visual system is going to assume great significance. It is probable that our life-span will reach before long its theoretical limit of about a century. Human self-destructiveness apart, the age-limiting organs are the nervous and vascular systems, the kidneys and the liver. We can survive without eye-sight. But this is true only individually. If a large proportion of older people were visually disabled the resulting social burden could be almost unsupportable. We have already noted that there are ethnic differences in the rate of aging and it is obvious that every effort has to be made to optimize our senile visual faculties if old age is to be made statistically more than bearable.

Questions

1(a) Given that the pupillary diameter varies inversely with the square root of age, show that the visual threshold for red light rises linearly with age.

 (b) Why is it necessary to stipulate the colour of the measuring light?

2   Give physical and physiological reasons for the differences, if any, between infant and adult visual resolution.

4 Perceptions

The previous chapters have dwelt on means rather than ends. We have considered a few of the mechanisms believed to be involved in transmitting visual impulses to our consciousness, sorting, selecting, simplifying, accentuating, concentrating on, features that may be wanted or needed; dove-tailing them into other sensory modalities, such as hearing, and marrying them to our memory when recognition is needed. And, if we are honest, there is only one reply to the question of 'How do we see?' It is, regrettably, that we do not know.

We can do what botanists and zoologists used to do centuries ago: we can classify our perceptions. We can divide them into colour and stereo-vision, into contrast phenomena, into various transient effects (cf. p. 152); we can even tabulate types of optical illusion (Robinson, 1972). But none of this has so far led to the flash of insight that 'explained' the course of the stars or the circulation of blood. Maybe the future will be more fortunate in this respect. The development of artificial intelligences may lead us to chance upon a concept which will make mental and, with it, visual activity intelligible. At present there are many sceptics who hold that mental processes cannot unravel an activity of their own kind. The question is whether, when we understand the behaviour of the major cellular assemblies of the brain, we can form a model with valid predictive properties. A system cannot be said to be understood until one's predictions about it are fulfilled on a statistically significant basis. The probability argument implicit in this approach recognizes the impossibility of taking into account every single cerebral cell of which there are 10^{10} or more.

There is little doubt that the probers in us seek to understand sensations and perceptions simply because we wish to understand understanding and, therefore, man. The key to man is his mind. But his mind reacts to the environment via senses of which vision is the one studied in greatest detail, not only because of its importance emphasized already by Aristotle, but also because the maturity of the physical sciences has made it amenable to quantitative enquiries which have yielded elegant relations. It is only fair to repeat (cf. p. 1) that the conditions in which visual systems are examined must be artificial if they are to be controlled. We know a great deal about the eye in the laboratory, but little of the eye in the field. In some respects this is disturbing. For example while there is a certain amount of comprehension of what is involved when we look at coloured tiddly-winks, the colour physiology of looking at Persian carpets or the kaleidoscope or psychedelic pictures is unexplored. No matter. It is not the job of a text such as this to be anything but retrospective: a simple stimulus gives rise to a sequence of events which probably represent one of the limiting sets of boundaries which a wider explanation will have to encompass.

Colour vision

Let us recall that, while the characteristics of small retinal areas (20′ in diameter and less) have been examined as regards their chromatic properties, the vast majority of studies has been concerned with test-fields approximately covering the fovea (< 1°).

This has isolated the rod-free area of the retina. We do not spend our time looking at such small fields. However, when larger, physiologically more meaningful fields, are studied, retinal areas are used which contain rods. The precise interaction between rods and cones is still a matter for debate (see p. 79), but, to make things more difficult, it varies appreciably e.g. with the luminance of the stimulus. These effects are, in turn, modified by the level of adaptation to which the retina is tuned.

In their static, physically abstract, state, four basic properties of the cone-mechanisms have received a great deal of attention, namely

(a) what is their sensitivity to radiations of different wavelengths?
(b) how readily is one wavelength distinguished from another?
(c) in what proportions are mixtures of matching stimuli composed so that a test-radiation may be mimicked in all respects? and
(d) what causes a break-down in the rules so established?

In view of the sensitivity of the rods, care has to be taken to ensure that they are excluded from the measurement when the sensitivity of the cones is being studied. This can be done in a variety of ways. Fixation of the eye and test-field size can be so arranged that only the rod-free part of the retina is stimulated. In theory, this can be done for a wide range of luminance levels. Another possibility is to adapt the eye to such a luminance level that the rods become saturated (p. 91). This occurs at approximately 200 cand/sq m, a level above which the cones are fully active and so amenable to study. The directional sensitivity of the receptors has also been used to separate the responses of the two systems, because that of the cones is significantly more marked than that of the rods (but see p. 20). Another type of segregation can be achieved by examining those abnormal observers whose rods do not function (nyctalopes).

Spectral sensitivity

When the spectral sensitivity (the reciprocal of the energy required to give a pre-determined response, perception, or sensation; p. 28) is determined with test-fields no greater than 50′ in angular diameter, the weighted curve due to a number of authors (Fig. 1.7) shows a maximum at 545 nm. This contrasts with the average curve standardized for photopic (i.e. cone) conditions obtained with fields which are greater than the rod-free area which peaks at 555 nm. Such curves must be independent of the nature of the source of light used in their determination. The energies recorded in the measurements are therefore computed for an equal-energy spectrum. If we want to compare the sensitivities e.g. with the absorption characteristics of the relevant cone pigments, it is necessary to convert the equal-energy correction into an equal-quantum one. Allowance for pre-retinal filters has already been mentioned (p. 6). Finally, if the effective pupil diameter is of the order of one third of a millimeter a diffraction correction is needed if great accuracy is required: in practice this will occur sometimes in connection with the Stiles–Crawford method mentioned on p. 20.

If the above tests are done not just with spectral test-fields, but with such fields seen against another spectral background, the curve of Fig. 1.7 becomes in general modified. The background is said to adapt the retina, notably those cones that are most sensitive to it. In general, this means that the modified curve represents the sensitivity of the more or less unaffected cone-groups. Fig. 4.1 shows a summary of such experiments which indicate that, broadly speaking, there are three independent cone sensitivity curves. Fig. 4.2 can be compared with these data: the absorbance measurements (p. 27) on single human cones are not inconsistent with the sensitivity data. But it has to be stressed that our understanding of light-absorption by objects with dimensions comparable with the wavelength of light is still incomplete, and a detailed comparison between the two categories cannot be pressed.

It may be mentioned parethentically that the individual curves of Fig. 4.1 may be modified in detail as a result of large luminance changes. This may be attributed as much to receptor changes as to neural modifications.

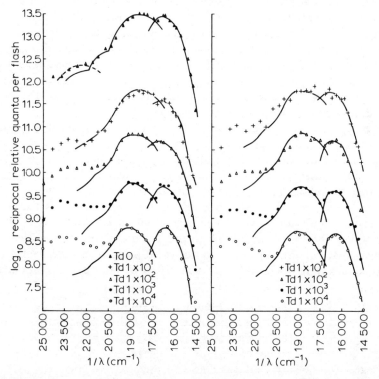

Fig. 4.1 Incremental spectral sensitivity of two observers for different retinal illuminances of a 5500°K background. The solid lines represent a theoretical function. The 0 troland curve (▲) on the left shows mean dark-adapted thresholds. Td, troland. (From Sperling and Harwerth, 1971. © 1971 by the American Association for the Advancement of Science.)

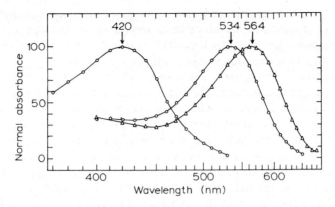

Fig. 4.2   The mean absorbance spectra of outer segments of the three classes of human photoreceptors. Curves labelled as follows: '420'–mean of three blue-sensitive cones; '534'–mean of eleven green-sensitive cones; '564'–mean of nineteen red-sensitive cones. (After Bowmaker and Dartnall, 1980.)

Colour matching

The triad of the cone mechanisms is met again in colour mixture. Photic stimuli can be mixed simply by projecting them on to the same retinal area. This is illustrated in Fig. 4.3. The sensation due to the test-stimulus (T) is that which it is desired should be matched by a suitable mixture of spectral stimuli λ_{1-3}. The optical superposition is achieved here schematically with three mixing cubes divided diagonally by semi-reflecting surfaces. The arrows indicate that the luminance of each matching stimulus is under independent control: the relative proportion of each is uniquely determined by T.

In theory, the three matching stimuli (on no account should they be called primaries as painters and psychologists are wont to do) can be derived from anywhere in the spectrum provided only that none of them can be matched by a mixture of the other two. If this proviso is obeyed then it will be found, within limits, that the whole visible spectrum can be matched by mixtures of three matching stimuli, varying only in their relative proportions. This is also true of non-spectral stimuli such as white. This generalization, known for well over two centuries, led Thomas Young (1802) to propound the trichromatic theory. It postulates that colours are perceived via three independent mechanisms. As biological cells were discovered only some 30 years later by Schwann and by

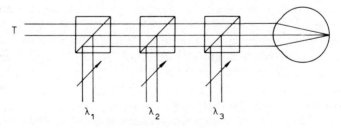

Fig. 4.3   Principle of light mixture.

Purkyně, it was not possible for Young to identify the residence of trichromacy. Clearly, the grouping of the absorbance spectra of individual cones in three spectral regions suggests that the locus is in the receptors, a feature in information transmission which economy would in any case demand.

It is convenient to represent the above proportions of the three matching stimuli in a diagrammatic form, which shares some features with Newton's colour circle. For example, it is possible to rationalize the energy units of the matching stimuli so that the values needed to match some standard white shall sum to unity. Then it suffices to plot the relative proportions of just two of the matching stimuli (MS), the third being obtainable by subtraction from unity. By convention the plot is presented in terms of a red and a green matching stimulus, as practical considerations call for red, green and blue MS's. The resulting chromaticity diagram (Fig. 4.4) shows that to match e.g. a test radiation of wavelength 540 nm, the proportions of R, G, B are 0.123, 0.901, − 0.024 respectively. Clearly, an intense test-light will need more of each MS, but, within limits, the proportions will remain constant. In practice, the shape of Fig. 4.4 changes at low luminance levels or when only non-foveal cones are being used.

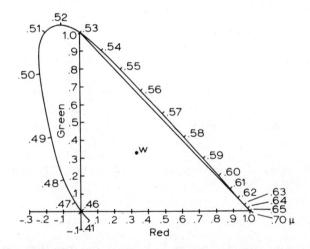

Fig. 4.4 The chromaticity chart using the matching stimuli 460, 530, 650 nm, but with their units adjusted to bring white W to co-ordinates 0.333, 0.333. (After Wright, 1946.)

Although we mentioned a standard white, this is something of an abstraction. In fact, Wright (1946) has shown that what we call white is literally coloured by our age: owing to the yellowness of the crystalline lens (p. 133) the apparent white point is moved in the direction of the chromaticity of its dominant wavelength, approximately 575 nm. The dominant wavelength λ(d) relates to test-stimuli with chromaticities inside the spectrum locus: these can be matched by a mixture of white and λ(d). This alternative means of specifying chromaticities is quantitatively equivalent to the previous one.

The discrimination of chromaticities is theoretically complicated because equal distances in the chromaticity diagrams do not correspond to equal sensory distances. There is no valid manner of measuring sensation magnitudes, and the sensory distances are expressed in terms of numbers of just discriminable chromaticity steps. These are small e.g. as between white and 570 nm: we say that this yellowish-green radiation looks desaturated in contrast with, say, 460 nm.

Wavelength discrimination

The size of step along the spectrum locus is of special significance. Known as the wavelength discrimination curve (Fig. 4.5), it represents the smallest change in wavelength the eye can discern at any spectral point. Note that the least changes occur at about 490 and 580 nm: under good conditions the eye will distinguish between equi-luminant areas differing by as little as some 2 nm.

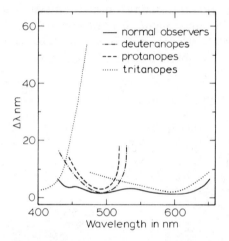

Fig. 4.5 Wavelength discrimination curves characteristic of the principal types of colour vision. (From Weale, 1960.)

Colour defects

However, this is not true of all people. In Western countries, there are about 2 per cent of all men, and a small fraction of a per cent of all women who consistently record larger steps than normal. Mostly this occurs predominantly at longer wavelengths (Fig. 4.5). This means in practice that they fail to distinguish red, green, yellow, and orange (of equal luminance). They are, therefore, referred to as red-green defective. The group as a whole can be further sub-divided, notably into those who have relatively little sensitivity to radiations of long wavelengths (protanopes) and those whose sensitivity is normal (deuteranopes). They are distinguished from the normal majority in that they can match the whole of the spectrum with just two matching stimuli whereas normally three are needed (see above).

A small number of people have analogous problems at the short-wavelength end of the spectrum and are known as tritanopes; they, too, are dichromats (Fig. 4.5). They confuse e.g. blue with yellow, and violet with pink even when the test-fields are relatively large. This stricture has to be made as even normal people make similar confusions with test-fields subtending areas as little as 15′ in extent. It has recently been demonstrated that the operative variable is not so much the size of the test-field but rather its spatial frequency Fourier transform, i.e. even normal people fail to resolve e.g. yellow/blue gratings of 4 or more c/°.

The colour-matching population is not made up only of di- and trichromats. A very small fraction consists of two types of monochromats, i.e. people who match the spectrum with only one variable stimulus. One type – cone monochromats – are normal in all other respects. But the other, namely rod monochromats, are characterized by reduced or zero cone activity, and consequently have poor visual resolution even in daylight.

Some 5 or 6 per cent, though trichromats, cannot be accommodated with the normal majority for the simple reason that neither group accepts the matches of the other. The cause of this is still unknown, hypothetical explanations ranging from postulates of anomalous cone pigments to anomalous chromatic processing. Not even monkeys whose colour vision appears to match ours in all respects have been able to clarify this age-long problem. Table 4.1 gives an approximate distribution of the incidence of colour anomalies in the West.

Table 4.1.   Approximate distribution of types of defect amongst males in Western Europe and white males in the United States.

Type	Percentage
Anomalous Trichromatism:	
Protanomaly	1.0
Deuteranomaly	4.6
Tritanomaly	0.0001
Dichromatism:	
Protanopia	1.2
Deuteranopia	1.4
Tritanopia	0.00004
Monochromatism:	
Rod	0.003
Cone	0.000001
Total =	8.2

There are suggestions to the effect that colour vision is not fully developed until after infancy, and that it diminishes systematically in old age. In view of the complicated nature of colour vision tests the former is hard to substantiate; and the progressive yellowing of the lens makes it difficult to confirm the latter. What is certain is that the red-green dichromacies are sex-linked, the principle of inheritance of the defect being that the whole of the phenotype's X-chromosomes has to be affected, the conditions being transmitted via one of its genes. The transmission of tritanopia being so much rarer, it remains to be seen whether it is, for example, autosomal, as has been claimed (Kalmus, 1965).

Contrast

At present, there is no remedy for colour defects. However, vocationally their handicaps are being progressively reduced, and in some forms of art, they are, it would seem, being turned to advantage. It is, of course, easy to be facetious about this. But a moment's reflection shows that there are important aspects of colour which have so far, received only a limited amount of serious study. From the point of view of art, and indeed from that of everyday life, contrast offers an important aspect.

Classically divided into two groups, namely simultaneous and successive, it is analysed thereby on a purely phenomenological basis. The former is the name given to the apparent change in colour neighbouring fields mutually induce in each other. Thus a bright red pencil or postage stamp placed on a neutral background gives it a greenish tinge. When the stamp or pencil is removed, the tinge vanishes from the background but appears in the area vacated by it: this is known as successive contrast.

As far as I know these effects have not been generally quantified rigorously, nor do we know the precise laws which relate them to retinal position, stimulus size, intensity, and duration.

On seeing blue

An important exception is provided by recent work done on the so-called blue-sensitive mechanisms (BSM) of the retina (cf. Fig. 4.1), the one believed to be inoperative in tritanopia or 'blue-deficiency'.

There are several peculiar problems associated with BSM. Even in the dark-adapted fovea it is the least sensitive of the retinal mechanisms (cf. Fig. 1.7). This is only partly due to the possibility that the number of blue-sensitive cones in the fovea is relatively low. For when one examines one's fovea with as nearly a violet point source as can be obtained with short-wavelength radiations there is never a time when, on moving a fixation spot, the point source appears to flash on and off. This is also true of red and green point sources which are visible throughout this part of the retina. But a firm conclusion is reached from studies of absorption measurements of individual cones: the relative proportions are connected with pigment characteristics as shown in Table 4.2.

When we consider the scarcity of blue-absorbing cones then their low apparent sensitivity is hardly surprising. The calibration of the energy used to measure

Table 4.2. The relative numbers of blue- green-, and red-sensitive cones and their relation to foveal sensitivity S

λ max	Transverse absorbance (A)	% population (P)	Effective cross section (A × P)	S	S/(A × P)
420	0.037	8	0.003	50.9	17
534	0.032	32.5	0.0104	81.3	7.8
564	0.027	59.5	0.0161	100	6.2

sensitivity evidently involves the whole of whatever test-field is used. But if the retina is 'patchy' insofar as mainly blue-sensitive cones are concerned then the radiation falling in between them is going to be wasted. The last column represents the ratio of columns 5 and 4 (Table 4.2) and shows that the low blue sensitivity is partly explicable in those terms. S has been corrected for the transmission characteristics of the crystalline lens (Fig. 1.5a) and of the macular pigment (Fig. 1.5b).

However, BSM appears to suffer from a second disability. The primate colour system seems to be organized on the basis of an 'opponent-colour' principle, traceable to the Prague psychologist Ewald Hering and, through him, to Goethe, the German poet. Briefly, once the receptors have processed chromatic information, hypothetically organized nervous pathways (p. 34) treat 'red' in opposition to 'green', and 'yellow' in opposition to 'blue'. The inverted comma notation is a shorthand indication of the spectral stimulus having led to the response under discussion. In practice, to quote one example, adaptation to one of a pair of opponents will facilitate stimulation of the other. There are other symmetries of this sort buttressing the concept at a post-receptoral level. A recently reported exception to this elegantly symmetrical scheme resides in the blue *enfant terrible*: adaptation of the human eye to yellow light raises the threshold for blue light but only after the adapting field has been turned off (Fig. 4.6).

The view held by a number of people is that blue-sensitive cones by-pass a data-processing stage available to red and green-sensitive receptors, and have access only to the 'opponent-colours' stage. Then BSM would be controlled not only by blue-sensitive but also by other receptor groups, active at longer wavelengths.

If, moreover, such an input were accompanied by an attenuation of the short-wavelength response, other 'blue' peculiarities may be easier to understand (Mollon, 1977). This is true even of anomalies in the colour sense, no matter

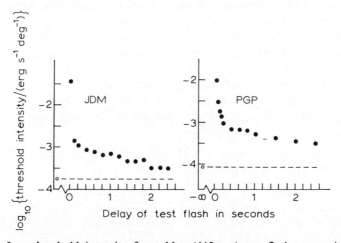

Fig. 4.6 Log threshold intensity for a blue (445 nm) test flash at varying delays following the offset of a yellow (580 nm) field of intensity $10^{-1.4}$ erg s^{-1} deg^2. o ---, incremental threshold when the field is present. Two observers. (From Mollon and Polden, 1977. © The Royal Society, London.)

whether these are acquired or inherited, and there are indications even in the extreme case of colour deficiency, namely cone-monochromatism, that post-receptoral anomalies may be more noxious than those at receptor level.

It is evident from the above outline of a rapidly changing field of study that our earlier view that the human fovea is blue-deficient is too circumscribed. The fovea, and perhaps also the retinal area surrounding it, is tritanopic for small stimuli. However, Mollon and Polden's experiment shows that there are important dynamic ingredients in the situation: clearly duration of exposure is a relevant consideration, and one not easy to control outside the laboratory when we recall that the eyes are subject to endless minute involuntary movements in addition to intended ones (Carpenter, 1977).

Colour and contours

This point is particularly significant in view of the fact that the relation between colour vision and stimulus configuration has received an impetus from an unexpected quarter. By realizing the very important role of contours, Celeste McCollough (1965) made one of the most far-reaching observations in the field of colour study. Suppose that a vertical grating on an orange background is viewed for a moment, and then the gaze is switched to a horizontal one of the complementary colour, namely blue-green. One's gaze is alternated in this manner for two to four minutes. If one then views the test shown in Fig. 4.7 an orange after-affect is seen on the right and a blue-green one on the left, provided colour-vision is normal. The effect is perceptual as turning the figure through 90° leaves the (desaturated) colours associated with the respective directions of the grating. The colour effects are therefore linked with hypothetical edge detectors, neurones of which have been identified by electro-physiological means (cf. p. 151). It may be mentioned parenthetically that the after-effects revealed by the achromatic gratings are not pure complements of the inducing stimuli. This is

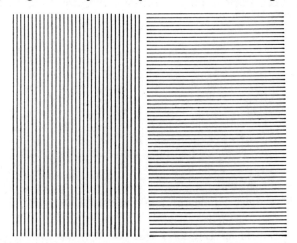

Fig. 4.7   Test pattern used in four orientations. After adaptation to orange-vertical and blue-green-horizontal, the left half appears blue-green and the right half appears orange when the pattern is shown as above. (After McCollough, 1965.)

possibly due to the fact that achromatic gratings can, at least in some observers, elicit chromatic effects without prior chromatic inspection. It seems, then, that the visual field is not radially uniform as regards the chromatic responses of edge detectors. These phenomena are seen best (if at all) with an achromatic grating having a spatial frequency of 3–4 c/° (but see below).

The question of whether the effects are to be associated with retinal or cortical neurones (or both) has been approached by stimulating the visual system binocularly and monocularly with a systematic variation of colour and grating direction. The colour sensations elicited subsequently by Fig. 4.7 depended on whether the grating was viewed binocularly or with each eye in turn. This would locate the responsible neurones in the cortex, but we shall see below (p. 148) that the evidence is less unambiguous when it comes to edge detection. Stromeyer (1972) and May *et al.* (1978) have stressed that the direction of the grating is not the only determinant: its spatial frequency plays also a role. For example with 0.8 c/° stimuli, the maximal effects (measured by colour matching) were obtained when one or more of the fundamental Fourier components were in the same orientation. On the other hand, at a higher frequency (3 c/°) they were observed when adapting stimuli had their fundamental Fourier components at 45° to each other. In other words, viewing distance can play a role in the chromatic perception that edge detectors may mediate.

One of the significant attributes of the above phenomenon is that, once it is established, it can persist for hours without further chromatic 'priming'. In particular, its duration far exceeds that of after-images which one can observe after viewing a high-contrast stimulus, no matter whether it is chromatic or achromatic. It is worth noting that the McCollough effect does not need fixation, whereas after-images are improved by it. Indeed, the McCollough effect is likely to be vitiate by fixation which can be shown to lead to perceptual image-fading, particularly when it comes to contours. This distinction was used in a colorimetric determination of the duration of both after-images and the McCollough effect, and extrapolations from Fig. 4.8 show that threshold purity

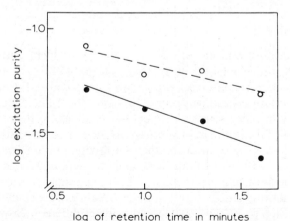

log of retention time in minutes

Fig. 4.8 Mean values for log excitation purity, combining magenta and green values, plotted against log time (in min) for McCollough effect (○). Negative after image (●). Best fitting lines by least squares are also shown. (After Hansel and Mahmud, 1978.)

values would be reached after 24 hours from the (negative, i.e. complementary) after-image, and 190 hours in the McCollough effect. The extrapolation may not be justified, but the difference between the two effects is evident and points to the involvement of different neurone populations.

The details of the underlying systems are still somewhat obscure. It is noteworthy, e.g., that the achromaticity of the test-pattern (Fig. 4.7) is not a *sine qua non*. If the usual pair of chromatic gratings is used for induction purposes, and the test-response is carried out on a pair of chromatic gratings, then it can be shown with colour matches of the latter that the McCollough effect is admixed to them. It is likely that there is nothing special in the orange/blue-green combination originally selected: the luminance of the stimuli coupled with their contrast probably contributed to the success of the original experiment. But the fact that the induced responses are additive to the direct ones exempts the specific spectral characteristics of the test: what matters is their differential effect on the retinal cones.

A qualitative explanation of the McCollough effect may be sought in the organization of the visual system. For example cells with receptive field characteristics earlier associated with X and Y cells (pp. 43–44) have been detected in the retina of the macaque monkey. Moreover, they exhibited opponent-colour responses. This concept, which is traced back to Hering (p. 145), implies that a response to a given spectral stimulus is paired, in opposing circumstances, with another, generally complementary stimulus. For example given a receptive field with an on-centre and off-surround, the system would work on the basis of green-centre, red-surround or *vice versa*, etc. X-cells are associated with such a system, whereas Y-cells would share the input for centre and surround from at least one type of cone even if, perhaps, to different degrees. This type of observation, if applicable to man, coupled with an elongated receptive field, would provide a framework for the McCollough effect on an adaptation basis. It is not the phenomenon as such that is complicated as the fact that its persistence is long.

Colour and size

When one is dealing with edges, another different problem arises. We have already noted that small retinal areas are tritanopic (p. 144). What is one to expect when a series of such colour-defective areas are juxtaposed and strung in a row? Rentschler (1973) suggested that the visual system adds the individual responses (not necessarily in a linear fashion). Now the smallness of the retinal area is defined in terms of the stimulus, or alternatively, in terms of its spatial frequency equivalent. Is it just a coincidence that sensitivity to short-wavelengths is relatively poor at high spatial frequencies *and* for small visual angles (p. 143)?

One way of approaching the problem is by using gradients of varying slopes defining the width of the above row of 'small' areas. This is another way of looking at blur (cf. p. 17). Two juxtaposed fields of different chromaticities (p. 141) are made to overlap gradually: if the region of overlap is narrow the gradient is said to be high and *vice versa*. Rentschler (1973) determined for three regions of the chromaticity diagram (Fig. 4.9) by how much the chromaticity has to be changed to render the blur region visible for different gradients. Two field sizes were used, namely 2.5° and 12.5° in angular diameter. Fig. 4.9 shows that there is a clear difference in the two sets of conditions. When the gradient is high (low width of blur region) the threshold chromaticity difference remains constant for blur widths approximately included in the fovea. As the width begins to exceed its diameter the threshold rises. In the case of the smaller field the rise starts without any hysteresis presumably because additivity plays a less important role than at 12.5°. Note also that, in the small field situation, there is a systematic variation from red to blue: once the 'tritanopic' width of blue is exceeded ($\sim$ 30′), a further reduction in the gradient causes the threshold to remain at a fixed level. The possibility that the spectral variation shown in Fig. 4.9 may have an optical (diffraction) component cannot be ruled out.

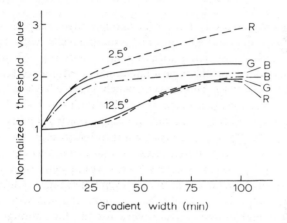

Fig. 4.9 Normalized threshold-blur functions for different colours and field sizes. (After Rentschler, 1973.)

The important notion that we may be colour-defective for chromatic contour regions has been elaborated with particular reference to non-spectral chromatic stimuli. It is possible to predict the visibility of chromatic borders successfully on the assumption that red- and green-sensitive cones provide an input into opponent colour neurones so that, if the luminances of the two half-fields forming the region of blur are kept constant, the distinctness of the border depends simply on the differential stimulation of those two cone populations. Since protanopes and deuteranopes have monochromatic vision in conditions in which the normal eye exhibits small-field tritanopia, their responses to chromatic borders are simpler than is true of trichromats. The reason is that they (probably) lack the red- and green-sensitive receptor systems respectively. A determination of the differential stimulation (in terms of energy units) of the red and green systems implies therefore that the sensitivity of one of the mechanisms is being charted, the stimulation of the absent one being zero. Within rather wide limits, this expectation is fulfilled.

Pointillism

There is a host of practical applications of these rather fundamental considerations. Colour appearance in textiles provides an example amenable to ready study, but there is no need for the suggestion that the phenomena just discussed are, in any sense, new. The presence of thick dark strips in the leaded glass of our mediaeval churches and in that of many continental cathedrals is sufficient proof that the problem of border chromaticity must have obstructed itself in its most insistent form in the only painting technique to be based entirely on scientific principles, namely pointillism developed by Georges Seurat, the French post-impressionist artist.

Seurat hoped to replace the subtractive process of mixing pigments with the optical additive mixture of lights reflected from minute adjacent areas painted on the canvas in conformity with Chevreul's 'laws' (1839) of contrast. This, Seurat believed, would lead to enhanced brightness. Since any one pigment gives rise to chroma by absorbing the complementary chroma from incident white light, the addition of pigments leads to more absorption: therefore less light is reflected from the surface. But if the pigments are juxtaposed instead of being mixed this loss is avoided. Pointillism relies on the failure of the eye to resolve small adjacent areas, and on the consequent 'optical' mixing of the various bundles of light coming from the elementary chromatic reflectors.

We shall see below why this superficially reasonable theory fails in practice. It was known to fail within a year or two of Seurat taking Paris by storm when he exhibited *L'après-midi d'un Dimanche à la Grande Jatte* (1884). Indeed, at an exhibition of his work in Brussels in 1889, the complaint was that his work looked grey and colourless. Seen from a distance of some ten metres, this is certainly true of *La Poudreuse* in the Courtauld Gallery, London. Homer (1964) gives a tortuous account of how the appearance of a pointillist painting changes with viewing distance. A very much simpler means of demonstrating the attendant colour changes is provided e.g. by a pair of opera-glasses used back to front. If one of the oculars is held in front of one eye, then one can compare the apparent colour change with the unaided eye: the minification through the ocular is equivalent to doubling or trebling the viewing distance. The inevitable drop in effective luminance can be compensated with a grey filter in front of the free eye.

The above remarks on small-field tritanopia and on borders indicate that the so-called scientific basis underlying pointillism is erroneous. Rooted as it is in 'laws' of contrast, if fails precisely because Seurat contrasted small, and not, large, areas. The proportion of border per unit (circular) area is much greater in small than in large areas. Moreover, the appearance of neighbouring coloured areas is reciprocally affected by their relative extents, chromaticity, luminance and so on. No rational system has yet been evolved from studies of even simple patterns. To speak of a scientific basis for a situation involving 'hundreds and thousands' is therefore at best premature.

The matter is consequently aggravated by the circumstance that, if Seurat followed a system on his palette, it was invalidated the moment he touched the canvas: on the palette the coloured areas were relatively large, but not so on the canvas. We saw above that the 'laws' of contrast are likely to differ in the two cases. Seurat's scientific misfortune was that Arthur König, in 1894, was the first man to write about the changed appearance of small coloured areas since the Roman author Lucretius. The Frenchman's tragedy was that König reported his observations five years after Seurat's untimely death.

We saw (p. 148) that, what has since come to be called foveal or small-field tritanopia is a problem linked to high spatial frequencies. Seurat's pointillism clearly creates a situation where it can operate beyond a certain viewing distance, so leading to colour confusion and loss of chroma. Daw (1968) has done some electro-physiological experiments on retinae of goldfish which throw further light on the problem. He either inserted a fine micro-electrode into the ganglion cell layer of the retina or else apposed it to an optic nerve fibre: these two procedures are equivalent as the fibres of the vertebrate optic nerve are merely the axons (processes) of the ganglion cells. He stimulated the retina with a small spot of light in order to establish the extent of the receptive field of the particular ganglion cell or nerve fibre (cf. p. 42).

Having mapped the relevant fields, Daw stimulated each of them e.g. with a central red spot (Fig. 4.10) and a surrounding red annulus in turn. The response produced by the red spot could be abolished by the simultaneous addition of a suitable annulus. But it was enhanced if the annulus was green. If the central spot was minute, the enhancement failed to take place. This is only to be expected, as the above-mentioned abolition of the response occurred also for a green centre and a green surround. Like centres and surrounds antagonise each other. A similar mechanism appears to operate also in human vision. A red disk surrounded by a green annulus appears with a more saturated red than when the

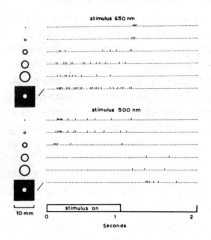

Fig. 4.10 Response of a goldfish retinal ganglion cell to various spots and annuli. Red light (top): 650 nm of irradiance 1.3×10^{10} quanta.mm^{-2}.sec^{-1}; green light (bottom series): 500 nm of irradiance 6.5×10^{9} quanta.mm^{-2}.sec^{-1}. Illuminated areas are shown black and non-illuminated areas white. Dimensions in the plane of the retina: diameter of spot 0.36 mm; diameters of annuli $0.72-1.08$ mm, $1.44-2.16$ mm, $2.88-3.60$ mm, $4.32-5.04$ mm and $2.16-10$ mm square. The stimuli are drawn approximately to scale opposite the responses which they elicited. (From Daw, 1968. © 1968 The Physiological Society.)

red disk is much reduced in diameter. This effect may be related to border, small-field, or high frequency tritanopia.

The plasticity of the various colour sensations as revealed in some of the above observations is an important indication of the fact that the popular association between a spectral band and the chromatic sensation it evokes is, at best, loose. That it may be altogether non-existent has been demonstrated by a number of authors. The most striking illustration is due to Gehrcke who showed, by varying the rate of rotation of disks, such as those shown in Fig. 4.11, that monochromatic (yellow) sodium light can produce the sensations of red and blue. The underlying mechanism depends probably on a number of facts: when a red car-braking light is imaged on the retina, especially in a non-foveal region, it may remain unnoticed until it is turned off. It then gives rise to an unmistakable blue-green sensation. Whatever processes of adaptation may be involved, a change in chroma from positive to zero can lead to an altogether different chromatic response. If the stimulus change is gradual the switch-over is not observed: thus the rate of change plays a material role, which may explain why Gehrcke's disks give rise to different sensations depending on the rate and sense of rotation. Thus a single monochromatic stimulus, suitably modulated, can act *as if* it were culled from a different part of the visible spectrum. Note that we appear to be dealing with an illusion only if we postulate a one-to-one relation between stimulus and response. Just as tears may be due either to a stimulus normally producing sadness or happiness, but the response is still tears, so a given chromatic response may occur as a result of different types of stimulation. This illustrates the care that has to be exercised when attempts are made to characterize responses and sensations in terms of stimuli that evoke them.

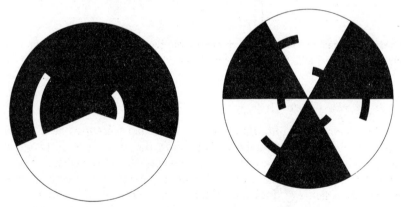

Fig. 4.11   See text. (After Gehrcke, 1948.)

Stereoscopic vision

Although stereoscopic vision differs from colour vision more than is true, e.g., of the sensation of light, the 'as if' situation can be found also in the space sense. Its function is to locate the relative fronto-parallel planes wherein different objects distributed 'in depth' may be found. It is therefore based on a metric lying in the sagittal plane, and on perpendiculars bisecting the distance between the two eyes.

When both eyes lead to single vision owing to the fusion of the messages initiated by the two retinal images (cf. pp. 39, 155), the fiction of the single, cyclopean eye is introduced, which locates this imaginary visual organ in the above sagittal plane.

Depth perception

Stereoscopic vision needs to be carefully distinguished from depth perception. The former depends on the use of both eyes, the latter may, but need not, do so. For example, in Fig. 4.12, the rectangular area A appears to be in front of the rectangular area B either in the bin- or the monocular mode. The side view shows, of course, that this is an as-if situation: not only is A behind B, but, in addition, neither area is a rectangle. Thus, while overlay is a clue to depth it is not a clue to stereoscopic vision and stereoscopic vision cannot be mimicked simply by overlay in the sense in which yellow light can be mimicked by a suitable mixture of red and green stimuli (p. 141). A number of other, so-called monocular, clues will occur to the thoughtful reader. They may be based on relative luminance, shape, colour, contour etc but, clearly, always involve a comparison between at least two points. Whereas we can say this spot is mauve or bright or minute, we cannot say it is behind without referring it to some other spot.

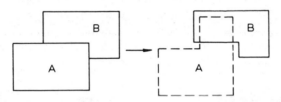

Fig. 4.12 The pair of superimposed figures on the left appear to represent two rectangles. The 'real' figure on the right shows only one of a number of possibilities as to what the truth might be.

Clues to stereo-vision

We shall see below that important clues to binocular stereopsis have recently come to light. But the oldest established of them is the disparity of the two retinal images. This is how it operates. If the head is kept still and each eye is closed in turn then, though the same view is before us, it appears slightly different depending on which eye does the looking. The nature of the difference (i.e. parallax) is clear as it can be mimicked by using only one eye and displacing one's head so that the eye occupies the position of its fellow and its own in turn. The distance of necessary displacement is equal to the interpupillary distance and amounts approximately to 63 mm.

However, there are limits to the degree of disparity which can induce stereo-vision. For example, if an object is well within the nearest distance of distinct vision (~ 30 cm), disparity is liable to become so great that fusion cannot be achieved even though the retinal images may be greatly out of focus. As an approximate guide-line, it may be taken that the ensuing images (double vision) are such that the difference between their superposition 'in register' would have an angular subtense in excess of the spatial resolution threshold in the relevant retinal region. However, as Helmholtz proved, a mere consideration of contours is insufficient: e.g., two parts of a stereogram viewed in a stereoscope (a device that ensures that each eye sees only one component as in a Viewmaster) give rise to a stereo-illusion. If one of them were replaced by its negative, the same pairs of contours would be present yet no stereo-illusion would ensue.

It cannot be argued that this is only to be expected because the fused figure would not make 'sense'. The question is whether the fused images would lead to a sensation since + and − sum to zero. Sense or otherwise does not seem to be relevant: e.g., the 'impossible' object shown in Fig. 4.13 gives rise to a stereo-illusion when viewed in a stereoscope. But the above negative-positive paradigm illustrates a type of competition between the two eyes, which is aptly called 'retinal rivalry'. The race goes some times to the left, at others to the right.

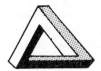 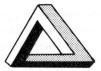

Fig. 4.13 'Impossible' stereo-effect. If the figure is held close to your eyes and gradually moved away, three triangles are seen with the centre one 'in depth'.

After-images

Insofar as the avoidance of retinal rivalry is a pre-requisite for fusion, it is remarkable that it is only relatively recently that our understanding of the problem has been advanced. One of the reasons is that, in the past, the effect of small eye-movements does not seem to have received sufficient attention. These occur all the time, even when we think that we are firmly fixating a definite spot in the visual field. Although the vast majority of eye movements are conjunctive, i.e. there is a high correlation between the directions and (torsional) senses of the left and right eye movements, disjunctive movements do occur. It is conceivable that these are maximized in the above positive-negative contour situation. This hypothesis can be tested e.g. when the retinal images are immobilized by suitable optical levers. There is, however, another method of studying properties of immobilized retinal images: this involves after-images.

As their name implies, after-images are perceived after a stimulus has been imaged on the retina. In practice this means also that they are perceived after the appropriate stimulus has been withdrawn. For a century or more they were studied as a phenomenon *sui generis*, and therefore largely by psychologists: but they may more properly be looked on as part and parcel of the physiological processes stemming from the normal stimulating processes, even though they are revealed more readily at high contrast.

The after-image is evidently fixed on the retina, its break-up and ultimate dissolution being due to normal restorative sequences which are unrelated to eye-movements even though the attendant blur suggests movement. Wade (1973) used after-images due to differently oriented gratings in a study of retinal rivalry and distinguished between their positive and negative appearances: the former is analogous to a positive print of a retinal image, the latter to its negative. With each of the above gratings flashed simultaneously respectively into each of the two eyes, rivalry occurs when one looks at a steady background. When however, the projection area of the after-images is illuminated intermittently, rivalry occurs when the after-images are positive, but fusion is perceived when they are negative. While the reason for this is obscure, it suggests further studies if for no other reason than that after-images must be generated even if they are not perceived: hence the existence of rivalry under normal conditions may be due to such latent processes.

In fact, Wade compared rivalry in the two situations: whereas both the duration and the frequency of dichoptic rival after-images varied with orientation, vertical gratings persisted for longer than was true of 45° ones; no such effect was observed for rival real gratings. More specifically, rivalry between real images is less prolonged than is true for after-images: it is undecided whether eye movements are responsible for this. This difference persists up to a point even when gratings are replaced by single lines, i.e. binocular rivalry is not influenced by orientation, and dominance periods for real lines are briefer than is true of after images.

Fusion

Although, as we shall see below, cortical cells for disparity detection have been recently uncovered, the mechanism for fusion is still obscure. We may, however, ponder whether, in searching for such a mechanism, we are asking the right question. Suppose that the visual system is organized to detect diplopia. Then, in the appropriate circumstances, failure of diplopia being detected will betoken the detection of fusion. We only seek a mechanism for fusion because we understandably consider it to be something desirable. To draw an analogy, when the dash-board shows no warning light in action, we assume all is well with the car: a mechanism of action will only start being revealed when the warning lights show up. Similarly, it may suffice for an understanding of fusion if the perception of diplopic images is elucidated.

Disparity

The absence of diplopia *per se* is insufficient for depth perception: disparity is also needed (but see below). Now the classical view of disparity is that the two retinae receive two images of the same object but that their sizes are different. This glib description almost always obscures the fact that the difference in size is confined to the horizontal dimension (Fig. 4.14a). This distinction between the horizontal and vertical scales is ignored of necessity also in the more modern approach which examines disparity in terms of differences between the two retinal images not as regards size but spatial frequency (cf. p. 11). Thus it can be shown that, if two

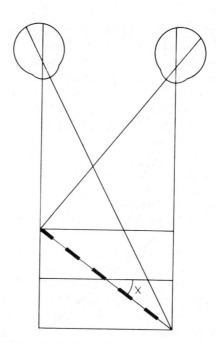

Fig. 4.14a The periodically thickened line represents a grating, tilted about its vertical axis by an angle X, being viewed binocularly. (After Blakemore, 1970.)

vertical gratings of different spatial frequency are presented one to each eye, conditions for fusion exist and the combined percept appears to be turned (Fig. 4.14b) about a vertical axis. The role played by contrast in this new type of stereophenomenon is as yet unresolved. This notion has been subtly elaborated by Tyler and Sutter (1979) who see the texture of surfaces as a more likely vehicle for information about spatial frequency differences than is to be found in different sizes. They postulate a stereo-mechanism based on 'diffrequencies' to be seen perhaps as an early evolutionary step toward disparity processing because the precision needed is smaller by an order of magnitude. The reason is that textured stimuli permit areal averaging which is more advantageous than the gauging of distances between vertical contours. A physiological substrate buttressing this attractive hypothesis awaits discovery, and may perhaps tie up with the sort of minute eye movements mentioned on p. 154. A recent model of stereo-vision which has not gone unchallenged, postulates the existence of different perceptual disparity channels characterized by a specific spatial frequency at which they operate optimally and which also determines the disparity range peculiar to each of them.

One feature of this concept relates to the initiation of vergence movements of the visual axes: channels tuned to low frequencies, i.e. those associated with large receptive fields (pp. 50–52) mediate vergence movements so as to achieve the binocular correspondence of more discrete receptive fields having a higher frequency response, i.e. being involved by textural detail. If it could be shown that hunting vergence movements are not random, the hypothesis would clearly be sustained.

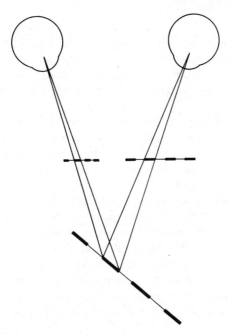

Fig. 4.14b A schematic representation of how the spatial disparity hypothesis can predict the sensation of depth. (After Levinson and Blake, 1979.)

Random-dot diagrams

One of the signal advances in recent research on stereo-vision is associated with the production of a stereoscopic sensation with contourless stimuli (Julesz, 1971). Two random-dot diagrams (Fig. 4.15) are produced by means of a computer and one is presented to each eye. Close inspection reveals that they are not entirely similar: the central area can be shown to be displaced laterally. When such a diagram is viewed in a stereoscope (p. 154) for about 20 seconds the central area clicks forward or backward depending on the phase of the displacement.

(a)   (b)

Fig. 4.15 When the diagrams are inspected monocularly they appear made up of random units. But when they are stereoscopically fused, a square is seen below a surround. (From Julesz, 1971.)

Stereo-geometry

The phase of more than one area can, of course, be displaced. A study based on such an arrangement was used to detect the afore-mentioned vergence movements, and it was shown that disparate textures can act as triggers for correct (i.e. non-random) vergence movements, and that stereopsis may be facilitated by them.

It is important to distinguish this concept of phase from that appertaining to the Fourier description of a stimulus. This appears to play an important role in the fusability of gratings capable of evoking stereoscopic sensations. For example, the harmonic content of gratings displayed on a phosphorescent screen can be controlled electronically (cf. p. 14). Levinson and Blake (1979) have compared the dichoptic presentation of gratings of similar spatial frequency but different harmonic content with other pairs which were both sinusoidal but differed e.g. by 10 per cent in spatial frequency. The former cannot be fused to evoke a sensation of depth, whereas the latter can (cf. p. 156). This new observation seems a little drastic in its implications: we may be faced with an all-or-none situation, but it is more likely that, when appropriate threshold experiments are carried out with a step-wise variation in harmonic content, the difference between the two situations will be found to be one of degree rather than one of kind.

In principle, such experiments involve a quantitative judgment of depth. It is only by adaptive modifications of stimuli that subservient mechanisms may be segregated. The geometry of the situation is simple (Fig. 4.16). Let a be half the inter-pupillary distance, with L representing the left eye. D is the distance of the nearer of two points lying in the sagittal plane SP. Let Δ be the smallest separation between them ($= PQ$) when the disparity for both eyes combined is $\theta - (-\theta) = \nabla$.

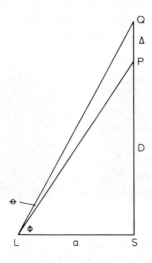

Fig. 4.16   The geometry underlying the concept of retinal disparity (cf. Fig. 4.14).

Then, since $\theta = \nabla/2$ and $\tan\phi = D/a$

$$(D + \Delta)a = (\nabla/2 + D/a)/(1 - D\nabla/2a)$$

whence it follows that $\Delta = \nabla D^2/(2a - \nabla D)$

Thus the minimum discernible depth Δ increases approximately with the viewing distance. Note that the threshold reaches infinity, i.e. stereoscopic vision vanishes when $D = 2a/\nabla$. Given that $2a \sim 64\,mm$, and a reasonable experimental value for $\nabla \sim 15''$, $D \sim 880\,m$. This is only another way of saying that, at large distances, the convergence of the visual axes becomes negligible: both retinal images then become similar in all respects.

In the above case, therefore, D would be kept fixed. Stimulus conditions would be varied so as to minimize Δ, with ∇ depending on the correct functioning of the observer's oculo-motor mechanism; in case of squint it will probably be abnormal. It is easy to see that the angle ∇ can be expressed in terms of frequency when the target is a periodic stimulus. While the above value of $15''$ is not atypical, Tyler (1977) has stressed in an instructive review that thresholds as low as $2''$ have been reported: this would imply that the observer's space discrimination extends to over 6 km. It has to be remembered, however, that disparity is a function of the size (spatial frequency) of the target. This is brought out in more detail in another study involving random-dot diagrams: whereas the random-dot pattern resolution was about 40 c/° (i.e. close to a resolving power of 1.5′), a stereo-grating composed from a pair revealed a maximum resolvable frequency of only 4 c/°: at low spatial frequencies monocular and stereoscopic resolutions are similar for comparable levels of contrast. This low stereoscopic band width implies e.g. that if it were ever practicable to broadcast television signals suitable for dichoptic- as distinct from binocular-viewing, this could be done within economic bounds in terms of the cost of bandwidth.

The ability to extract overall stereoscopic information from such 'noisy' stimuli is likely to be achieved if two parts of the brain can scan the two images and peel out their relative disparity. Work on cells responding to disparate stimuli has recently been reviewed by Zeki (1979) who based his study on the following considerations.

Cerebral pointers

A point moving from a to b appears to move in opposite directions in the two eyes (Fig. 4.17). We noted that the cortex contains binocularly driven cells. If, amongst them, there were such as to respond specifically e.g. to two edges moving in opposite directions, one in each eye, they might provide a basis for a disparity mechanism. Such cells occupy areas V2, V3 and V3A, and the response of one found in the posterior bank of the superior temporal sulcus has the required characteristics (Fig. 4.18). Such cells may be differently sensitive for slits and for edges, and a monocularly driven cell cannot respond unambiguously: how does it distinguish a movement in depth from a change in apparent size (cf. p. 49)? The answer seems to be that it does not have to do this as it does not operate on its own. Although one monocular cell can be foxed in this manner, binocular stimulation leads usually to an out-in response via one eye and an in-out response via the other. If the target is a long way off the sagittal plane, both eyes may signal

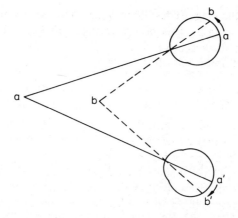

Fig. 4.17 Diagram to show that when a point a, having its images at a and a′, is displaced to b, having its images at b and b′, the displacement is in opposite directions in the two eyes. (From Zeki, 1974. ©1974 The Physiological Society.)

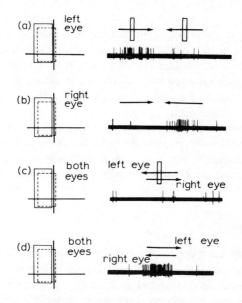

Fig. 4.18 The response of a cortical cell in the posterior bank of the superior temporal sulcus to stimulation of the two eyes of a monkey. The receptive field for the ipsilateral (right) eye is marked by the broken rectangle, that for the contralateral eye by the solid one. (a) Stimulation of the contralateral eye by a slit of light moved in the directions marked by the arrows; (b) the same for the ipsilateral eye; in (c) the response to simultaneous movement in the null directions (i.e. those giving no response) for each eye is shown; (d) the response to simultaneous movement of a slit of light in the preferred direction for each eye is shown. Duration of each trace was about 5 s. Receptive field was $4\frac{1}{2}° \times 2°$. (From Zeki, 1974. © 1974 The Physiological Society.)

a similar sense but the magnitudes differ. When both sense and magnitude are similar, differentation fails. This occurs in the retinal periphery presumably because the sizes of the receptive fields (p. 52) are too large (or high spatial frequency discrimination is cut off).

Dynamic effects

Although stereo-acuity, like monocular acuity, is maximal in the fovea, non-foveal parts sometimes play a role that is still unclear. The Pulfrich phenomenon is a case in point. When a pendulum is binocularly observed in a fronto-parallel plane (Fig. 4.19), and a filter of neutral density (~ 0.5, cf. p. 27) is held in front of one eye, most people observe a peculiar phenomenon which, like the random-dot images, takes some time to build up. The pendulum is perceived to be moving in a horizontal plane. However, rigid fixation of the pendulum or too small an angular subtense greatly weakens the effect, if it does not altogether vitiate it. An interaction between target and background is also observed in a stationary stereo-situation: e.g. contours flanking a stereo-target lead to a significantly reduced acuity for depth to be recorded, especially if the contours are presented 100 ms after presentation of the test. As eye-tracking movements involved in following the moving pendulum reveal 'hiccoughs' of comparable duration, the two observations may be linked. The elementary explanation of this illusion was advanced by the one-eyed Pulfrich: the eye provided with the filter has a longer latent period than is true of the other. Consequently the message the brain receives from it is older than is true of the bare eye (but see below). Hence the two eyes project the origins of corresponding messages to lie along a locus that may be a wide ellipse, a circle, or a long ellipse, depending on stimulus parameters. The theory is verified within limits, but there are problems associated with distortions

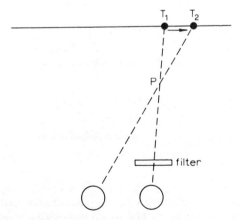

Fig. 4.19 The Pulfrich phenomenon. If the right eye is partly occluded with a grey filter and an object moves from left to right, the unoccluded left eye sees it more quickly than does the right one. The brain projects T_1 and T_2, the two points in time of seeing, to the intersection of the visual axes (P). When the sense of movement is reversed, the axes appear to intersect behind the horizontal line. The locus of P is an ellipse with its axis behind $T_1 T_2$. (From Weale, 1968.)

in the apparent trajectories and it leaves out of account the existence of hypothetical mechanisms that are concerned with the looming appearance of approaching targets (see below).

Although the phenomenon is illusory in the sense that the pendulum bob moves virtually linearly, it is accompanied by an interesting objective corollary. It is possible to record eye-movements not only video-or cinematographically but also electrically. The reason is that the eye behaves as if it were a dipole, with a positive charge on the cornea. If a couple of electrodes are attached to the skin near each eye then the movement of the charge during an eye-movement can generate a recordable voltage. Movements of less than 1° have been recorded in this way, which is by over an order of magnitude less sensitive than e.g. photo-electric techniques, but adequate for our purpose. When such an electro-oculographic record is made of an observer following a Pulfrich target the eyes are found to converge and diverge as though the illusion were real, (Reading, 1973). This is a remarkable variant of kinaesthetic impulses, a system of messages informing various parts of the body of the activity of others. We may note in passing that, as convergence of the visual axes is reflexly accompanied both by accommodation and pupillary miosis (p. 132), it would be interesting to know whether they, too, accompany the Pulfrich illusion. This might provide a useful pointer for the study of nervous pathways involved in this peculiar phenomenon.

We may also note parenthetically that in one of the notorious so-called ambiguous figures, the Necker-cube (Fig. 4.20), which involves unreal planes of projection because it can be interpreted with the plane ABCD being either in front or at the back, no change in accommodation can be established when perceptual reversal occurs.

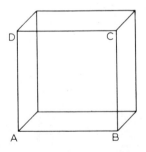

Fig. 4.20   Necker Cube

A recent study has shown that the Pulfrich phenomenon cannot be due just to the two eyes recording messages dating from different points in time respectively. Burr and Ross (1979) observed two spots of light each moving on one oscilloscope screen stroboscopically in such a manner that the left eye saw its spot a time δt before the right time saw its own: consequently the two targets cannot have been seen by the two eyes in two different positions at any one time. The spatial separations and the period of presentation were chosen so as to render their movement apparently smooth. The virtual disparity ∇ between the two targets, given by $\delta t \times \Delta/\tau$ led to a stereo illusion when ∇ exceeded 3 seconds of arc or about 200 μs. It is, of course, conceivable that, both in this experiment and in the Pulfrich effect, it is not the stimulus that primarily evokes the illusion, but rather a cellular memory affected differentially. Clearly, the experiments share the notion of dichoptic delay, but differ as regards continuity of stimulation. But if this difference lies more in the stimulus than in the physiological response then we shall have to wait for experiments on a monkey's disparity detectors in order to be certain that delay and disparity are equivalent and interchangeable stimulus parameters.

From a biological point of view, there is a significant difference between position in depth on the one hand and motion in depth on the other. It is not often appreciated that the latter can be ambiguous. For example, it is not always easy to decide at a glance in which sense a rotary garden sprinkler, raised to eye level, is in fact turning. In this case perspectival clues are useless, contrary to what would be true of a solid rotor (but see below). But the ambiguity can also be observed with solid objects. Often on winding, rolling roads it is not possible immediately to decide whether a vehicle is moving toward or away from us if we look purely along a horizontal line (Fig. 4.21). This notion is a generalization of what Helmholtz described as the Windmill illusion. When a windmill (or the above rotor) is seen merely as a silhouette against the sky with the plane of rotation including a small angle with the line of sight, the sense of rotation of the vanes can be ambiguous if the stereo-clues are very weak. In our ancestral past, such an ambiguity might have given an advantage to an escaping hunted beast, and it may well be that zigzaging hares and rabbits have evolved their indirect run just for this purpose.

The sensory mechanisms dealing with this problem have been studied in detail only recently (for a review see Regan *et al.*, 1979). The underlying optics which translates physical motion in a sagittal (depth) direction into imaged motion approximately perpendicular to it along the two retinal surfaces is easily derived

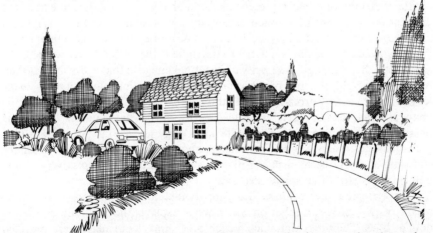

Fig. 4.21 When we are on the same level as the traffic there are situations when directions of motion may be confusing. In the above situation we may be undecided as to whether a large vehicle (further away) is coming towards us, or a nearer smaller one is driving away from us.

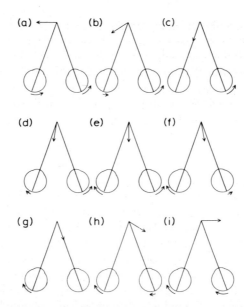

Fig. 4.22 Relative velocities of the left and right retinal images of an object provide a cue to the direction of motion of the object in depth. For example, if the left and right images of the object are moving in the same direction (a, b, h, i), the object will pass wide of the observer's head, whereas if only one image is moving (c, g), the object will hit the observer directly in one eye, and if the images are moving in opposite directions at the same speed (e), it will hit him directly between the eyes. In addition, if the left image is moving more slowly than the right one, the object will pass closer to the left than to the right eye, and if the right image is moving more slowly, the object will pass closer to the right eye than to the left eye. (After Regan, Beverley and Cynader, 1979.)

from a consideration of Fig. 4.22. In this figure two points are shown in different sagittal locations: they may represent an object or alternatively, the same object at different points in time (this notion of movement is generalized in Fig. 4.17). In (a) an object moves horizontally, parallel to the line joining the eyes: its retinal image moves with equal (angular) velocities to the right. If the object moves wide off the left eye (b), then the angular velocity of its retinal image in that eye is smaller than is true on the right; clearly if the object moves along the line joining it to its image (c), the image velocity drops to zero. In this context we can ignore the fact that the image *size* increases at a maximal rate. The rest of the Figure covers 180° of the possible velocity vectors, the other 180° involving merely a change in sign. This raises the question of whether the relative angular velocities might not perhaps stimulate a stereo-mechanism sensitive to such a stimulus irrespectively of any binocular disparity that might also exist.

In experimental tests of these ideas, apparent stereo-motion was produced by means of two television tubes on which were displayed horizontally oscillating dots or lines. The tubes were facing each other and the displays were reflected from semi-reflecting surfaces (Fig. 4.23) placed in front of the observer at the centre of the arrangement. Suitable alignment of the two optical paths vis à vis the eyes created the illusion as if a fused image of the two tube-screens were formed on a cyclopic screen, and, depending on the directions of the movements, the displays could be made to appear to move forward or backward.

To begin with, the stereoscopic sensation was strong. However, after a few minutes it faded, suggesting that the visual system was becoming adapted to it. As no such adaptation appeared to mere side-ways motion (when the reflected images of the tube displays moved in the same direction), a specific mechanism was very probably in action. Indeed, as shown in Fig. 4.24, the adaptative

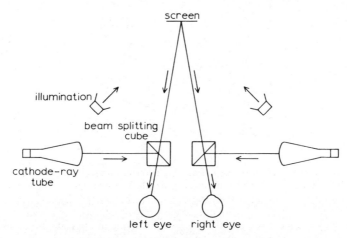

Fig. 4.23 Independently moving stimuli such as bars, rectangles or fields of dots were generated on a pair of cathode-ray tubes and presented separately to an observer's left and right eyes. The fused stimulus (here a rectangle) appeared against a white square on the screen opposite the observer. When the stimuli for the two eyes were made to oscillate in opposite directions, the fused stimulus seemed to be moving in depth along a line passing between the eyes, and when the stimuli were made to oscillate in the same direction, the stimulus seemed to be moving in depth along a line passing wide of the head. (After Regan, Beverley and Cynader, 1979.)

mechanism varies with the angle of the vector shown in Fig. 4.22. The continuous curve shows how the minimum detectable oscillation varies with this angle: the sensitivity for the symmetrical situation is relatively low (the oscillation needed for detection is 6 min of arc), but drops as the ratio of the velocities approaches a maximum (cf. Fig. 4.22 above). Then the observers were adapted for 20 minutes to a target moving apparently toward the left of the nose. When the original measurements were repeated the dashed curve was obtained. The converse (dotted curve) was obtained for adaptation on the right.

The number of such tuned channels is not large: specific adaptive angular segments are four in number, each comprising two opposite directions of motion. Their angular widths w vary enormously which is the reason for the peculiar abscissal scale in Fig. 4.24: channels operating 'between' the eyes have w's of some 1.5° whereas the others cover the remainder of the angular range.

It might be thought that the illusion of movement in depth is accompanied by one in size. Early in the fifties there appeared a series of studies on the apparent variation in size of the Pulfrich pendulum bob. The common-or-garden observer

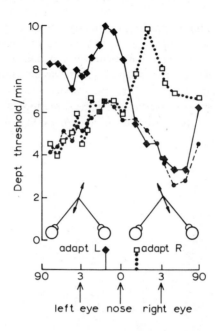

Fig. 4.24 Evidence for directionally selective stereoscopic motion channels. Threshold amplitudes of 0.8 Hz disparity oscillations are plotted against the equivalent real-space directions of oscillations.--, before adaptation; ——, after adaptation at L; . . . . , after adaptation at R. The small insets illustrate the L and R adaptating directions. (From Regan, Beverley and Cynader, 1979.)

is so taken aback by the unexpected stereo-*movement* that the stereo-magnitude of the image frequently passes unnoticed (see also below). But there is a noteworthy paradox: the pendulum bob appears to be larger when it is distant than when it is near. It may be that this is a manifestation of nothing more than a parallel of Emmert's observation – dubiously honoured as a 'law' – according to which a percept such as an after-image has an apparent size proportional to the distance of the surface whereon it seems to be projected. Consequently, a given bob moving in an apparent, i.e. unreal elliptical or circular trajectory will appear with a periodically varying size.

In its more contemporary form, a size variation can be detected in the type of experiment shown in Fig. 4.24. More specifically, an after-effect is observed which manifests itself as an apparent change in size, measurable by a null method, wherein the illusion observed is cancelled by the observer. Now this effect was found to decay, as is true of the pure stereo-illusion, as mentioned above. However, the rates of decay of the two phenomena are, in the ratio of about 4:1 (Fig. 4.25) which suggests that different neural mechanisms underlie the two effects. The rapid decay of the size-effect may explain why relatively few people become aware of the size variation of the Pulfrich bob.

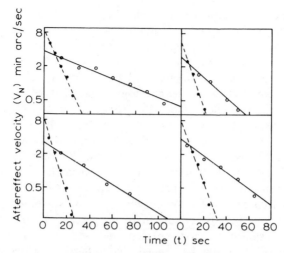

Fig. 4.25 Decay curves of the motion-in-depth after-effect and the changing-size after-effect for four observers. Nulling rates of movement of the vertical edges of the stimulus (V_N) are plotted logarithmically as ordinates vs the elapsed times after the cessation of adaptation (t) plotted linearly as abscissae. The decay of the changing-size after-effect is shown as the dotted line through the filled circles: the decay of the motion-in-depth after-effect is shown as the continuous line through the open squares. (After Beverley and Regan, 1979.)

Illusions

It is clear from the above account of illusionistic phenomena associated with stereo- and colour stimulation that some are part of 'the system'. Because they and others like them originally baffled the mind, they were frequently studied by psychologists who explained them in terms of perceptual concepts, rather than demonstrable mechanisms, just as I did above in seeking support from Emmert's Law: after all, what is a surface on which something appears to be projected, but actually is not? We must not be hard on experimental psychological researchers on this score: physicists did the same when postulating the existence of the luminiferous ether, and more recently, chemists hypothesized enzymes and catalysts without necessarily being able to isolate them.

However, it would be foolish to lump together everything that goes under the designation of illusions. Some like the above cube of Necker (Fig. 4.20) are trivial and, possibly linked to given cultural backgrounds (see below); others, like the impossible figures on p. 154 are just trivial; and yet others may be able to throw light, if not on visual processes themselves, at least perhaps on what is going on in the back-rooms behind the 'seens'. The latter are uniquely private: even if two people claim to have (had) the same vision, provided they have not communicated together, they are most unlikely to describe it similarly to a third person. In the opinion of the majority of people, any one hallucination is unlikely to be veridical, and, if experienced by more than one person, they will differ from one to another. Not so with illusions. Although not veridical either – whence their designation cognate with game or toy – they are usually perceived so uniformly as to be amenable to meaningful measurement. It is true that not all phenomena are perceived by everyone equally or at all, but the usual inference is that differences in the visual mechanisms, development or cultural background may account for variable data.

Measurement of illusions presents problems in certain circumstances. For example in the case of the Müller-Lyer illusion (Fig. 4.26), which exists in many forms (Robinson, 1972), the distance ab appears to be larger than bc. A ruler shows them to be equal. Now it is a fundamental scientific principle that, for a measurement to be valid when made more than once, it has to be made under comparable conditions. This does not happen in this case. The plastic ruler measures the length of the horizontal lines between the mere apices of the arrowheads, whereas the visual ruler uses the whole arrowheads. It is easy to devise a photo-electric measuring system which produces an objective illusion, i.e. measures ab as larger than bc without involving perception. In this instance, we apply the term illusion even so to the percept because of the almost blind faith we have in scales; but it could be argued that different metrics apply to the measurement of those horizontal straight lines, depending on whether or not arrowheads are present and detected: if they are not detected then they are not present as far as the sensor is concerned.

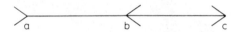

Fig. 4.26   Müller-Lyer illusion.

A second problem relates to the measurement of the magnitude of the illusory perception. The scale of the misjudgment in Fig. 4.26 can be determined, it is said, by moving the central arrowhead so as to make ab appear equal to bc. This is symbolized by ab ~ bc. It is arguable to what extent such a procedure measures the magnitude of the original illusion which has, in fact, been abolished so that the measurement might be made. As the two segments now appear to be equal, it is the plastic ruler that is suffering from an illusion. There is some merit in preserving the percepts of geometrical illusions and to measure their magnitude by appropriate matching techniques wherein the apparently modified components are matched by distortions when the perturbing factors are absent. On this view the Müller-Lyer illusion is measured more aptly by presenting an observer with lines ab and bc of various lengths and asking him to select a pair that matches those with fins.

This apparently facile argument is more substantial than might appear at first sight. There are various stimulus configurations that create illusions. The daughter vs mother (Fig. 4.27) is a well-known example. Why does it work? Its ambiguity depends on the absence of certain vital items of information: if what appears to be the old woman's nose were reddish as it is liable to be in older people then the alternative reading of Fig. 4.27 would be much harder. If the illustration were three-dimensional, misreading would be impossible (but see p. 163). That lack of information can lead to illusory situations is a matter of common experience as when one drives the car into a gate-post because of insufficient illumination. Mimicry and camouflage offer examples of ambiguity being created not by the absence of information but its surfeit. We see therefore that there is nothing absolute in a measurement such as the above, and that the notion of a ruler exhibiting an optical illusion is not so far-fetched after all.

The above-mentioned psychological approach e.g. to the problem of the Müller-Lyer illusion rests on a consideration of culture. When seen vertically, the

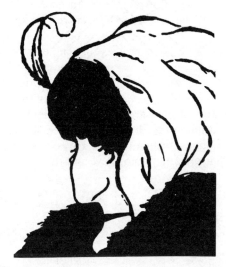

Fig. 4.27   Mother or daughter? (From Mütze, 1958. After W. E. Hill, 1915.)

segment ab is read as an internal corner e.g. of a room, while the segment bc would be seen as an external one, in analogy with concave and convex surfaces. Owing to a hypothetical scaling faculty, our perceptual system judges ab to be larger than bc because the pair of fins attached to the former make it appear to recede and vice versa. But if a more distant and a nearer line appear to project equal retinal images then the former must in fact be larger, which is how it is seen. As there is experimental evidence both in favour and in opposition to this interpretation, the question has to be left open. But as there are numerous other perceptual phenomena that seem to depend on cultural background, we shall do well to keep the possibility before us. For example, Eskimos that were brought up in igloos fail to see the above type of illusion because they have not been reared in a carpentered world. Similarly, there is some evidence that a rural population may be more susceptible to illusions involving perspectival clues because, at any rate in the United States of America, they may be more exposed to wide vistas than is true of urban dwellers.

Purely geometrical, as distinct from interpretational, illusions can also be classified operationally in the following manner:

i Those that are (Müller-Lyer) and those that are not (Zöllner, Fig. 4.28), observed when separated into component parts and presented as random-dot

170   *Perceptions*

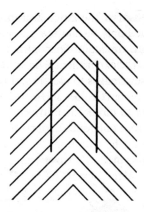

Fig. 4.28   Zöllner illusion.

stereograms (cf. p. 157). Thus when the fins are presented to one eye and the horizontal lines to its fellow the illusion is observed: its seat is therefore on the central side of the optic chiasma (p. 41). However, when the herring-bone pattern in Fig. 4.28 is presented to one eye and the parallel lines to the other,

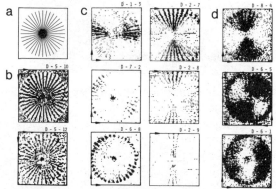

Fig. 4.29   (a) stimulus pattern: transfer patterns of neurones in the lateral geniculate body (b) and of cortical cells with (c) small and (d) large excitatory receptive fields. The stimulus pattern was $25° \times 25°$, scanned at a speed of 5–$6°$/s along vertical and/or horizontal parallel scanning paths in random succession across the receptive fields of the neurons recorded. The scan direction is indicated by arrows at the corners of the transfer patterns. The dimensions of the patterns in the scan direction represent time (5–6 s per scan path), but as the position of the transfer pattern relative to the neuronal receptive field is known at any moment, the time dimension is equivalent to space coordinates. Dots appear in the transfer patterns when the cell discharges during the scan procedure. A high dot density indicates a strong response to a feature of the stimulus pattern. The stimulus and the transfer patterns are aligned (or superposed, in later figures). (b) Top: transfer pattern of an on-centre cell in the LGB: the rays of the star are bright on a dark background (contrast 1.5 log units). Bottom: off-centre cell in the LGB, dark star on bright background. (c) cortical cells with small excitatory receptive fields. All cells except D-6-8 at the bottom of the left-hand column may be called simple cells, D-6-8 is hyper-complex. (d) complex cortical cells with large excitatory receptive fields. For the cortical cells, the stimulus pattern was always a bright star on a dark background. (From Creutzfeldt and Northdurft, 1978. © 1978 Springer-Verlag. New York.)

the illusion of non-parallelism of the latter disappears (cf. Julesz, 1971).

ii Illusions that are maintained only when their component parts are co-planar as distinct from those that are maintained also when this is not the case (Fig. 4.30). Note that from the experimental point of view two methods have been used to separate printed images to illustrate this. Julesz (1971) employed stereo-dot diagrams: by having red and green sets and providing the reader with a red and a green filter to place one in front of each eye he ensured that each eye transmits to the brain only one set of stimuli. Gregory, in 1970, used similar filters; he coloured the herring-bones in Fig. 4.28 red but the parallel lines green. Note that the two methods are not equivalent because Julesz does not allow us to use high spatial frequencies (cf. p. 11) which have been shown to be essential for the generation of some of these illusions.

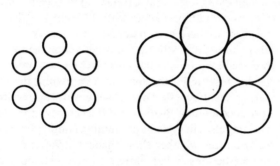

Fig. 4.30   Titchener circles.

This has to be considered in connection with the above classification which is concerned in part with the site of the phenomena, and *a priori* there is no case for assuming that there is only one. On the contrary, insofar as several authors have suggested that local inhibitory forces are at play (Carpenter and Blakemore, 1973), these may well act at either the retinal or the cortical level or at both. The fact that acute angles appear to be subjectively overestimated has been known for almost a century. A fairly plausible hypothesis suggesting that it may be due to inhibition occurring between orientation sensitive neurones has been put forward and tested by Carpenter and Blakemore. These neurones have been each shown to be tuned to a limited angular sector within which a stimulus can elicit their response. The basic assumption is that each neurone has a broad excitatory sector but is inhibited over a wider sector by neurones with identical and similar preferred responses. Two lines forming the flank of an angle of a few degrees will stimulate neurones interfering with each other's response such that the more proximal receptive fields will act in an inhibitory way, and the projected images will be splayed out in relation to their optical counterparts.

On the face of it, this hypothesis helps to account for a number of illusory effects, including the Zöllner illusion (Fig. 4.28). But the difficulty is that the neurones are located in the cortex (p. 46) whereas dichoptic viewing of the stimulus pattern abolishes the illusion both for low and high spatial frequencies, the latter being essential for the phenomenon: if Fig. 4.28 is looked at with poor focus e.g. at a distance without glasses correcting for myopia or shortsightedness, then the illusion vanishes even though all the lines may be visible. However, it can be perceived essentially only if both the perturbing and the perturbed elements appear in the same eye (see above). This does not invalidate the above hypothesis but raises the question of whether or not the primate retina or the cortical area 17 may not also contain an orientation sensitive system of sorts. It will be recalled (p. 47) that the fusion of two dichoptic inputs is unlikely to occur peripherally to area 18.

The Müller-Lyer illusion (Fig. 4.26) has recently been 'explained' also in terms of the above-mentioned overestimate of acute angles. Within certain limits, the magnitude of the illusion varies with the product of the length of the fins and the cosine of the angle they include with the horizontal, i.e. with the projection of the fins on the lines under comparison. It is plain that, if this is a valid explanation, equally long lines terminating in arrowheads subtending with the lines different angles should appear to have different lengths. This crucial experiment does not seem to have been described. Moreover, the Müller-Lyer illusion is observed dichoptically, whereas another phenomenon, the Zöllner effect, also believed to be based on angular mismatching, is not, as we have just noted. Now the paradox resulting from this is more apparent than real as more than one type of analysis has shown that neural networks, endowed with a short-term memory, can produce angular distortion if the activity of the neurones can be inhibited by lateral impulses in systems containing shunts. From our point of view it does not really matter whether these theories are rigorously correct in their explanation and predictions. What matters is the fundamental concept they allow us to examine.

We ask ourselves what is the essential difference, if any, between the retinal image as imprinted on the retinal rods and cones by the radiation absorbed in their outer segments on the one hand, and the corresponding spike potentials that can be picked up in the cortical cells on the other? In the past, we have been so obsessed in looking in the brain for what we find in the eye (Fig. 4.29) that, time and again, we overlooked the difference between a photograph and a perception. The path via networks, however, discourages the point-to-point approach (cf. p. 35). It reveals the meaning of pattern. A pattern involves significant repetition. Two of a thing can hardly be said to make one as they could be due to chance. But a few or more is different. However, a sensor, unlike a photographic plate or even the layer of rods and cones, cannot respond to the notion of a pattern unless it can make point-to-point comparisons. Note that whereas above the term point-to-point was used centripetally, i.e. in a hierarchic sense, now we use it collaterally, on one level. Such a comparison can be achieved successfully only with an elementary memory: the sensor must be able to respond to the image of some spatial element with 'I have responded like this two, three, etc. times before'.

It should now be clear why the earlier doubt about the relativity of some optical illusions (p. 168) may not be so far fetched. In several instances they are revealed when a comparison is made between (lateral) point-to-point metrics on the one hand, and net-work metrics on the other. Pattern cognition has to be distinguished from contrast cognition, and the higher faculty that it entails may have to be paid for in terms of non-linearity that is revealed as an illusion.

There are also trivial illusions, one or two of which we shall consider briefly because they have caused some misunderstanding. We have already met the impossible triangle (p. 154). A three-dimensional version of Fig. 4.13 has been produced (cf. Robinson, 1972), and presented as a surprising phenomenon. Now it will be clear after a moment's thought that the appearance of the monocular paradigm can be achieved only from one predetermined point of view (cf. Fig. 4.12). Theoretically, viewing has to be monocular with the active pupil occupying that point. The latter is defined so that the three-dimensional object presents the fixed two-dimensional projection which the uniplanar impossible triangle occupies on the printed page.

This and other impossibilities have appeared in various guises, but their existence is based on well-defined circumstances. One of these is the combination of eye-movements with a short-term memory, perhaps the type referred to above as essential for pattern cognition. If, as we scan the triangle, we did not remember at one corner what we saw at the previous one there would be no paradox. And the latter arises simply from a build-up of expectations: any two sides of the triangle lead us to expect the third to conform with them. The confounding of the expectations creates the paradox. We would be quite wrong to look on this as a purely visual effect. It is well-known to musicians. For example the phrase of a tune composed in G-major can end in D: but the chord accompanying the terminal note can be based on B-flat major since D figures in both scales. Much the same effect appears in a phrase such as 'The fact of the matter is made up of atoms of different weight a second thought has to be given to the fact of the matter . . .' It is aggravating nonsense resulting from expectations and associations being set up by one group of words, and altered by the next.

The multiple sensory modality of such tricks illustrates not visual processes (as is true e.g. of the Zöllner-group of illusions) but rather a perceptual inertia, probably essential for economy in the act of thinking. This activity would be frustrating if there were nothing that one could take for granted.

Illusions in art

We shall now turn to an aspect of illusions which does not always receive the attention that it seems to me to deserve. This is the fact that, for much longer than science can be said to have existed, they were used, not as a drawing-room entertainment nor even to indicate that our eyes can deceive us, as is true of the Zöllner illusion first described by Montaigne (trans. Hazlitt, 1842), but as a deliberate ingredient in both art and architecture. It is noteworthy that they tend to fulfil two very different functions in these disciplines respectively. Leaving aside Op Art for the moment, optical illusions may be said to have been used in painting to promote the notion of fashionable realism whereas in architecture they subserved deception by concealment. There is a difference. In the former, every device that mimics the three-dimensional world of light, shadows, colour, depth, and contrast is called into service to overcome the barriers offered by a two-dimensional surface. The acme of this illusion is achieved in the genre of *trompe l'oeil* when we are uncertain whether we are looking at a painting or 'the real thing'. In practice, such illusion requires the artist to be in consummate control of monocular clues to depth perception (p. 153), and also to realize that the apparent size of objects may be affected by others in their proximity. The Titchener Circles (Fig. 4.30) are an interesting academic example, and the moon illusion a fascinating practical one: both the sun and the moon seem very much larger near the horizon than near the zenith, a phenomenon long known to perceptive artists both in the West and the Far East.

It is difficult to be certain in a number of cases whether artists were consciously familiar with some of the observations described by experimental psychologists during the last century or two, but, in the case of the effect described by Mach in 1865 there is no doubt: this original discovery can be antedated in both painting and verbal description by well over three centuries.

Mach showed that if two juxtaposed uniform surfaces are seen reflecting different amounts of light (Fig. 4.31) the border between them appears to be

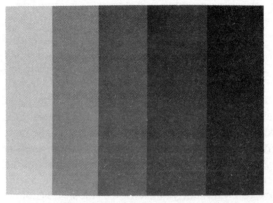

Fig. 4.31   Mach bands.

lighter than the light area on the side of the latter, and vice versa. The effect is said to be more easily observed when the transition between the two areas is less than sharp, and was attributed already by Mach to lateral interaction between adjacent retinal areas. This has been confirmed in numerous studies, not just on vertebrate retinae: the phenomenon subserves a mechanism that enhances contrast. The reverse, known as the Craik-Cornsweet illusion has also been observed: if a uniformly luminous surface is divided by a real luminance gradient that mimics the perception of a Mach-band then the two parts so formed appear to have different luminances. The apparently higher luminance goes with the brighter part of the border. It is noteworthy that the Mach effect was clearly and accurately described by Leonardo da Vinci in 1508, and had been painted even earlier by the Venetian Andrea Mantegna who had probably told Leonardo about it at the turn of the century. Ever since then Mantegna-bands have been a distinctive feature of Venetian painting, appearing in this country a century before Mach when Canaletto came here and painted the Thames and St. Pauls.

With the Florence of the Renaissance being universally accorded pre-eminent rank in its intellectual approach to the arts and sciences, the above and other contributions of more cosmopolitan Venice have come to be overlooked. Yet an architectural jewel of hers, the church of S. Maria dei Miracoli, was endowed with an illusionist exterior (Fig. 4.32), designed to provide impressiveness for what is a very small building. One of the tricks adopted by the Lombardi brothers who designed it is based on Brunelleschian perspective (cf. p. 173): by placing windows asymmetrically within niches, an illusion is created of the wall being much thicker than in fact it is. It serves to conceal smallness. If there were a lot of space surrounding the building then the design would be counter-productive from certain directions: but Venice being a high building-density area, the device has proved most effective.

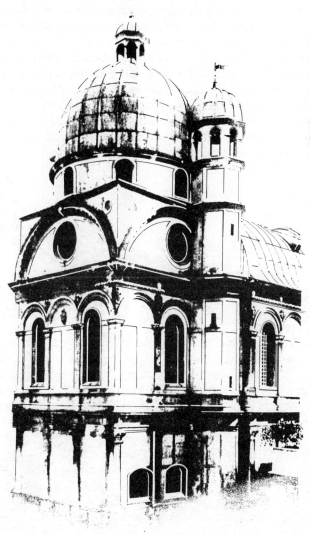

Fig. 4.32 The Church of S. Maria dei Miracoli, was furnished with an illusionist exterior, designed to provide impressiveness for what is a very small building. One of the tricks adopted by the Lombardi brother who designed it is based on Brunelleschian perspective (cf. p. 173): by placing windows asymmetrically within niches, an illusion is created of the wall being much thicker than in fact it is.

It is unlikely that the above example would have been realized in the absence of the discovery of the principles of perspective by Brunelleschi and, earlier, by Cavallini who, in their different ways, enabled painters to extend the pictorial power of the plane surface (see above).

However, architects, then more concerned with the appearance of buildings than they are now, also explored the use of illusions. This was in the best traditions of the trade. The Medici-Riccardi palace in Florence is clad with rusticated stones (Fig. 4.33). A three-storey building, its apparent height is exaggerated by the simple device of the rustication being cut less deeply at the upper floors. As we associate resolution of less detail with greater distance, we are led to infer a greater height from the absence of fine detail. This is, of course, another example of a treatment of surface by illusionist means and may be associated, in a sense, with painterly devices. But the Greeks showed, in their hey day, that they were aware of some of the effects under discussion, and this is revealed in some of their architecture, none of their paintings having survived.

From the physiological point of view, two are of particular interest in that they are manifested in several of their Doric temples (Paestum in Italy and the Parthenon in Athens), and therefore their discovery is datable to the fifth century BC.

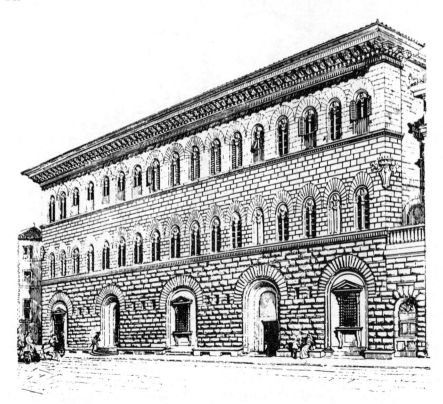

Fig. 4.33 The Medici-Riccardi Palace in Florence. The cladding of the wall gets more refined with height; this enhances the impression of height, especially when one looks upward. (After Fletcher, 1961.)

The first of these relates to the thickness and disposition of the outer columns of the naos, the colonnade surrounding the temple proper. The spacing is such that the distance between the corner columns and their neighbours is between 20 and 30 per cent smaller than is true of the other intercolumnar distances. The corner columns are also a few per cent thicker than is true of the others. Architects maintain that these features are designed to compensate for what they call the colour effect (Fig. 4.34).

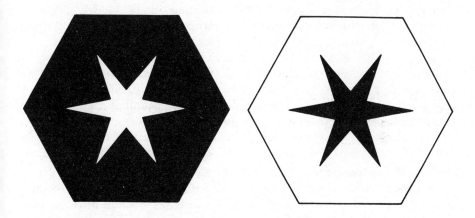

Fig. 4.34   The classical size illusion.

This misnomer – the effect is basically achromatic – is the name they give to what physiologists refers to as retinal irradiation. A dark surface on a light background generally appears to be smaller than an equally large light surface on a dark background. The effect which has been measured only recently (Fig. 4.35), varies with the relative contrast of the two fields, and, even at its largest, amounts to less than 10 per cent. Let us see how this may apply to the Greek temples. The idea is that, seen from its front, the row of columns appears against the dark background of the temple wall. But the corner columns are elevated against the light background of the sky seen through the naos. Without the above-mentioned compensation, the corner columns would appear to be thinner than the others and the corner spacing would appear to be too large. It is clear that the increase in columnar girth is in quantitative agreement with the data shown in Fig. 4.35, but the reduced spacing seems to overcompensate. Its explanation may therefore have to be sought on a different basis.

The other optical illusion involves the departure from verticality of the columnar axes. They are so inclined as to converge toward a point about 1.5 km above ground level. We noted on p. 171 that acute angles tend to be overestimated: hence obtuse ones appear to be smaller than they are. This means operationally that, if observers are asked to match such angles, they do so with smaller angles.

Now when one looks centrally up at the front of a building, one is looking into obtuse angles both on the left and the right. They are judged to be smaller than in fact they are. Consequently the building appears to be wider at the top than near

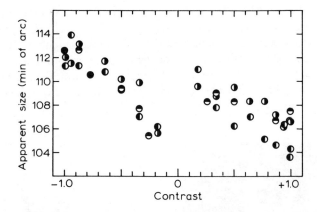

Fig. 4.35   Ordinate: apparent size of a square when covered with a diffusing screen so that its edges appeared blurred; abscissa: contrast (+ : dark on light). Angular subtense of comparison square 109′. Three observers. (After Weale, 1975.)

the bottom – a phenomenon easy to verify on most rectangular sky-scrapers such as the London Hilton Hotel or the New York Trade Centre. One way of reducing the apparent increase in width is, therefore, to increase the obtuse angles so that the building 'looks right'. The Greeks may consequently be credited with having been aware of a perceptual result of the hypothetical inhibition between orientation mechanisms believed to operate in our visual system. We may well ask with the sage whether there is anything new under the sun.

Questions

1 A stereo-illusion results when two different spatial frequencies are viewed dichoptically and fused. How and why is this related to the magnitude of the Pulfrich effect?

2 In about 1820, Turner painted a number of oil and water colour paintings in three colours in the belief that vision is trichromatic. Why was his theory in error?

3 Colour vision is affected by rod activity when the eye is in the mesopic state. Does this invalidate trichromatic matches? If so, how?

4 In chromatic stereoscopy, a red and an equally luminous, but separate, blue disks are presented on a black background. To many many people the red disk appears to advance and the blue one to recede. Why is this and how do you explain the exceptions?

Bibliography

The pages on which references occur are indicated by numbers in *italic*

Chapter 1

ARDEN, G. B. (1977). Three components of the photocurrent generated in the receptor layer of the rat retina. In *Vertebrate photoreception* (ed. H. B. Barlow and P. Fatt). Academic Press, London and New York. *33*

ARDEN, G. B. and ERNST, W. (1970). The effect of ions on the photoresponses of pigeon cones. *J. Physiol.*, **211**, 311–39. *33*

ARDEN, G. B. and LOW, J. C. (1978). Changes in pigeon cone photocurrent caused by reduction in extracellular calcium activity. *J. Physiol.*, **280**, 55–76. *33*

ASHMORE, J. F. and FALK, G. (1977). Dark noise in retinal bipolar cells and stability of rhodopsin in rods. *Nature (Lond.)*, **270**, 69–71. *29*

AZUMA, K., AZUMA, M. and SICKEL, W. (1977). Regeneration of rhodopsin in frog rod outer segments. *J. Physiol.*, **271**, 747–59. *27*

BOETTNER, E. A. and WOLTER, J. R. (1962). Transmission of the ocular media. *Invest. Ophthal.*, **1**, 776–83. *6*

BORNSCHEIN, H. and GUNKEL, R. D. (1956). The effect of rate of rise of photic stimuli on the human electroretinogram. *Amer. J. Ophthal.*, **42**, 239–43. *30*

BRIN, K. P. and RIPPS, H. (1977). Rhodopsin photoproducts and rod sensitivity in the skate retina. *J. Gen. Physiol.*, **69**, 97–120. *29, 34*

CALDWELL, J. H. and DAW, N. W. (1978). New properties of rabbit retinal ganglion cells. *J. Physiol.*, **276**, 257–76. *43, 44*

CAMPBELL, F. W. (1960). Correlation of accommodation between the two eyes. *J. Opt. Soc. Amer.*, **50**, 738. *17*

CRESCITELLI, F. and DARTNALL, H. J. A. (1953). Human visual purple. *Nature (Lond.)*, **172**, 195–6. *28*

DANIELS, J. D., NORMAN, J. L. and PETTIGREW, J. D. (1977). Biases for oriented moving bars in lateral geniculate nucleus neurons of normal and stripe-reared cats. *Exp. Brain Res.*, **29**, 155–72. *41*

DAVANGER, M. (1975). The suspensory apparatus of the lens. The surface of the ciliary body. A scanning electron microscopic study. *Acta Ophthalmologica*, **53**, 19–33. *18*

DE MONASTERIO, F. M. (1978 a). Properties of concentrically organized X and Y ganglion cells of *macaque* retina. *J. Neurophysiol.*, **41**, 1394–417. *43*

DE MONASTERIO, F. M. (1978 b). Center and surround mechanisms of opponent-color X and Y ganglion cells of retina of *macaques*. *J. Neurophysiol.*, **41**, 1418–34. *43, 44*

DE MONASTERIO, F. M. (1978 c). Properties of ganglion cells with atypical receptive-field organization in retina of *macaques*. *J. Neurophysiol.*, **41**, 1435–49. *45*

DOWLING, J. E. (1967). The organization of vertebrate visual receptors. In *Molecular organization and biological function* (ed. J. M. Allen). Harper and Row, New York. *23, 25*

DOWLING, J. E. and BOYCOTT, B. B. (1966). Organization of the primate retina: electron microscopy. *Proc. R. Soc. Lond. B.*, **166**, 80–111. *34, 35*

DRATZ, E. A., GAW, J. E., SCHWARTZ, S. and CHING, W-M (1972). Molecular organization of photoreceptor membranes of rod outer segments. *Nature New Biology*, **237**, 99–102. *26*

182   *Bibliography*

DRATZ, E. A., MILJANICH, G. P., NEMES, P. P., GAW, J. E. and SCHWARTZ, S. (1979). The structure of rhodopsin and its disposition in the rod outer segment disk membrane. *Photochem. Photobiol.*, **29**, 661–70.   25

EMSLEY, H. H. (1955). *Visual optics* (vol. 1.). Hatton Press, London.   5

ENROTH-CUGELL, C. and ROBSON, J. G. (1966). The contrast sensitivity of retinal ganglion cells of the cat. *J. Physiol.*, **187**, 517–52.   43

FOERSTER, M. H., VAN DE GRIND, W. A. and GRÜSSER, O. -J. (1977 a). Frequency transfer properties of three distinct types of cat horizontal cells. *Exp. Brain Res.*, **29**, 347–66.   43

FOERSTER, M. H., VAN DE GRIND, W. A. and GRÜSSER, O. -J. (1977 b). The response of cat horizontal cells to flicker stimuli of different area, intensity and frequency. *Exp. Brain Res.*, **29**, 367–83.   43

FRISÉN, L. and FRISÉN, M. (1976). A simple relationship between the probability distribution of visual acuity and the density of retinal output channels. *Acta Ophthalmologica*, **54**, 437–44.   39

FRY, G. A. (1955). Blur of the retinal image. *Brit. J. Physiol. Optics*, **12**, 130–52.   17

GALLOWAY, N. R. (1967). Early receptor potential in the human eye. *Brit. J. Ophthal.*, **51**, 261–4.   31

GOLDSTEIN, E. B., and BERSON, E. L. (1970). Rod and cone contributions to the human early receptor potential. *Vision Res.*, **10**, 207–18.   30

GREEN, B. H., MONGER, T. G., ALFANO, R. R., ATON, B. and CALLENDER, R. H. (1977). Cis-trans isomerization in rhodopsin occurs in picoseconds. *Nature (Lond.)*, **269**, 179–80. 25

HAGINS, W. A., PENN, R. D. and YOSHIKAMI, S. (1970). Dark current and photocurrent in retinal rods. *Biophys. J.*, **10**, 380–412.   32

HALL, M. O., BOK, D. and BACHARACH, A. D. E. (1969). Biosynthesis and assembly of the rod outer segment membrane system. Formation and fate of visual pigment in the frog retina. *J. Mol. Biol.*, **45**, 397–406.   25

HELMHOLTZ, H. (1855). Über die Accommodation des Auges. *Arch. f. Ophth*, **1**, Pt. 2, 1–74.   4, 17

HOLDEN, A. L. (1977). Responses of directional ganglion cells in the pigeon retina. *J. Physiol.*, **270**, 253–69.   42

HONIG, B., GREENBERG, A. D., DINUR, U. and EBREY, T. G. (1976). Visual pigment spectra: implications of the protonation of the retinal Schiff base. *Biochemistry*, **15**, 4593–9.   29

HSU, H. P. (1970). *Fourier analysis*. Simon and Schuster, New York.   11

HUBEL, D. H. and WIESEL, T. N. (1962). Receptive fields, binocular interaction and functional architecture in the cat's visual cortex. *J. Physiol.*, **160**, 106–54.   45, 46

HUBEL, D. H. and WIESEL, T. N. (1977). Ferrier Lecture. Functional architecture of macaque monkey visual cortex. *Proc. R. Soc. Lond. B.*, **198**, 1–59.   41–9

KAPLAN, M. W., DEFFEBACH, M. E. and LIEBMAN, P. A. (1978). Birefringence measurements of structural inhomogeneities in *Rana pipiens* rod outer segments. *Biophys. J.*, **23**, 59–70.   23

KAWAMURA, S., TOKUNAGA, F. and YOSHIZAWA, T. (1977). Absorption spectra of rhodopsin and its intermediates and orientational change of the chromophore. *Vision Res.*, **17**, 991–9.   24, 27

KNOWLES, A. and DARTNALL, H. J. A. (1977). In *The eye* (vol. 2B: *The photobiology of vision*) (ed. H. Davson). Academic Press, London and New York.   26

KOLB, H. (1970). Organization of the outer plexiform layer of the primate retina: electron microscopy of Golgi-impregnated cells. *Philos. Trans. R. Soc. Lond. B.*, **258**, 261–83.   35, 38

LATIES, A. M. (1969). Histological techniques for study of photoreceptor orientation. *Tissue and Cell*, **1**, 63–81.   7, 19

LATIES, A. M. and ENOCH, J. M. (1971). An analysis of retinal receptor orientation. I. Angular relationship of neighboring photoreceptors. *Invest. Ophthal.*, **10**, 69–77. 20

LE GROS CLARK, W. E. (1949). The laminar pattern of the lateral geniculate nucleus considered in relation to colour vision. *Docum. Ophthal.* **3**, 57–64.   40

MAFFEI, L. and FIORENTINI, A. (1973). The visual cortex as a spatial frequency analyzer. *Vision Res.*, **13**, 1255–67. *51*

MAFFEI, L. and FIORENTINI, A. (1977). Spatial frequency rows in the striate visual cortex. *Vision Res.*, **17**, 257–64. *52*

MARSHALL, J. and GRINDLE, C. F. J. (1978). Fine structure of the cornea and its development. *Trans. Ophthal. Soc. U.K.*, **98**, 320–8. *3*

MISSOTTEN, L. (1974). Estimation of the ratio of cones to neurons in the fovea of the human retina. *Invest. Ophthal.*, **13**, 1045–9. *35*

OPPEL, O. (1967). Untersuchugen über die Verteilung and Zahl der retinalen Ganglienzellen beim Menschen. *Albrecht v. Graefes Arch. Klin. Exp. Ophthal.*, **172**, 1–22. *38*

ØSTERBERG, G. (1935). Topography of the layer of rods and cones in the human retina. *Acta Ophthalmologica*, **13**, Suppl. 6, 1–102. *19*

OSTROY, S. E. (1977). Rhodopsin and the visual process. *Biochim. Biophys. Acta.*, **463**, 91–125. *28*

PHILLIPS, S. and STARK, L. (1977). Blur: a sufficient accommodative stimulus. *Doc. Ophthal.*, **43**, 65–89. *17*

READING, V. M. and WEALE, R. A. (1974). Macular pigment and chromatic aberration. *J. Opt. Soc. Amer.*, **64**, 231–4. *7*

RICHARDSON, T. M. (1969). Cytoplasmic and ciliary connections between the inner and outer segments of mammalian visual receptors. *Vision Res.*, **9**, 727–31. *23*

RIPPS, H. and WEALE, R. A. (1976). In *The eye* (vol. 2A of *Visual function in man*) (ed. H. Davson). Academic Press, New York and London. *9, 22*

RODIECK, R. W. (1973). *The vertebrate retina.* W. H. Freeman, San Francisco. *32*

ROHEN, J. and MRODZINSKY, K. (1955). Kerngrössenänderungen in der Netzhaut nach Belichtung. *Klin. Monats. für Augenheilk.*, **23**, 36–44. *36, 37*

ROHEN, J. W. and RENTSCH, F. J. (1969). Der konstruktive Bau des Zonulaapparates beim Menschen und dessen funktionelle Bedeutung. *Albrecht v. Graefes Arch. Klin. Exp. Ophthal.*, **178**, 1–19. *16*

STARK, L., TAKAHASHI, Y. and ZAMES, G. (1965). Nonlinear servoanalysis of human lens accommodation. *IEEE Transactions on Systems Science and Cybernetics*, Vol. SSC-1, No. 1, pp. 75–83. *18*

VAN ESSEN, D. C. and ZEKI, S. M. (1978). The topographical organization of rhesus monkey prestriate cortex. *J. Physiol.*, **277**, 193–226. *53*

WARWICK, R. (ed). (1976). *Eugene Wolff's anatomy of the eye and orbit* (7th edn.). H. K. Lewis, London. *40*

WÄSSLE, H., BOYCOTT, B. B. and PEICHL, L. (1978). Receptor contacts of horizontal cells in the retina of the domestic cat. *Proc. R. Soc. Lond. B.*, **203**, 247–67. *35, 37*

WEALE, R. A. (1958). Retinal summation and human visual thresholds. *Nature (Lond.)*, **181**, 154–6. *19*

WEALE, R. A. (1968a). *From sight to light.* Oliver & Boyd, Edinburgh and London. *2, 21*

WEALE, R. A. (1968b). In *Techniques of photostimulation in biology* (ed. B. H. Crawford, G. W. Granger and R. A. Weale). North-Holland Publishing Co., Amsterdam. *22*

WEALE, R. A. (1971). On the birefringence of rods and cones. *Pflügers Arch.*, **329**, 244–57. *24, 31*

WEALE, R. A. (1976). Ocular optics and evolution. *J. Opt. Soc. Amer.*, **66**, 1053–4. *36*

YOSHIKAMI, S. and HAGINS, W. A. (1971). Light, calcium, and the photocurrent of rods and cones. *Biophys. J.*, **11**, 47a. *33*

ZEKI, S. M. (1978 a). The cortical projections of foveal striate cortex in the rhesus monkey. *J. Physiol.*, **277**, 227–44. *53, 55*

ZEKI, S. M. (1978 b). The third visual complex of rhesus monkey prestriate cortex. *J. Physiol.*, **277**, 245–72. *55*

ZEKI, S. M. (1978 c). Uniformity and diversity of structure and function in rhesus monkey prestriate visual cortex. *J. Physiol.*, **277**, 273–90. *54, 55*

Chapter 2

ANDERSON, D. H., FISHER, S. K. and STEINBERG, R. H. (1978). Mammalian cones: disc shedding, phagocytosis, and renewal. *Invest. Ophthal. Vis. Sci.*, **17**, 117–33.   *84*

ARDEN, G. B. and WEALE, R. A. (1954). Nervous mechanisms and dark-adaptation. *J. Physiol.*, **125**, 417–26.   *71*

ASCHOFF, J. (1963). Comparative physiology: diurnal rhythms. *Ann. Rev. Physiol.*, **25**, 581–600.   *58, 61*

ASCHOFF, J. (1976). Circadian systems in man and their implications. *Hospital Practice*, **11**, 51–7.   *62, 63, 76, 78*

ÁSCHOFF, J., FATRANSKÁ, M., GIEDKE, H., DOERR, P., STAMM, D. and WISSER, H. (1971). Human circadian rhythms in continuous darkness: entrainment by social cues. *Science*, **171**, 213–5.   *67*

BASINGER, S., HOFFMAN, R. and MATTHES, M. (1976). Photoreceptor shedding is initiated by light in the frog retina. *Science*, **194**, 1074–6.   *87*

BESHARSE, J. C., HOLLYFIELD, J. G. and RAYBORN, M. E. (1977). Photoreceptor outer segments: accelerated membrane renewal in rods after exposure to light. *Science*, **196**, 536–8.   *85, 88*

BROWN, F. A. (1959). Living clocks. *Science*, **130**, 1535–44.   *58*

BRUCE, V. G. (1965). Cell division rhythms and the circadian clock. In *Circadian clocks* (ed. J. Aschoff), pp. 125–38. North Holland Publishing Co., Amsterdam.   *65*

BÜNNING, E. (1973). Light effects. In *The physiological clock* (3rd edn.). English Universities Press, London.   *60, 61*

DÖRING, G. K. and SCHAEFERS, E. (1950). Über die Tagesrhythmik der Pupillenweite beim Menschen. *Pflügers Archiv.*, **252**, 537–41.   *80*

DOTY, R. W. and KIMURA, D. S. (1963). Oscillatory potentials in the visual system of cats and monkeys. *J. Physiol.*, **168**, 205–18.   *59*

GLOSTER, J. (1966). *Tonometry and tonography*. J and A Churchill, London.   *57*

HARPER, D. W. and ZUBEK, J. P. (1976). Changes in critical flicker frequency during prolonged visual deprivation. *Perception and Psychophysics*, **19**, 551–4.   *77*

HOFFMANN K. (1965). Overt circadian frequencies and circadian rule. In *Circadian clocks* (ed. J. Aschoff), pp. 87–94, North Holland Publishing Co., Amsterdam.   *61, 62*

KAPPERS, J. A. (1976). The mammalian pineal gland, a survey. *Acta Neurochirurgica*, **34**, 109–49.   *72, 73*

KNOERCHEN, R. and HILDEBRANDT, G. (1976). Tagesrhythmische Schwankungen der visuellen Lichtempfindlichkeit beim Menschen. *J. Interdiscipl. Cycle Res.*, **7**, 51–69.   *78–80, 91*

KRIEGER, D. T., KREUZER, J. and RIZZO, F. A. (1969). Constant light: effect on circadian pattern and phase reversal of steroid and electrolyte levels in man. *J. Clin. Endocr.*, **29**, 1634–8.   *75*

LA VAIL, M. M. (1976). Rod outer segment disk shedding in rat retina: relationship to cyclic lighting. *Science*, **194**, 1071–4.   *85, 86*

LOBBAN, M. C. (1965). Dissociation in human rhythmic functions. In *Circadian clocks* (ed. J. Aschoff), pp. 219–27. North Holland Publishing Co., Amsterdam.   *64*

MEDDIS, R. (1968). Human circadian rhythms and the 48 hour day. *Nature (Lond.)*, **218**, 964–5.   *65*

O'DAY, W. T. and YOUNG, R. W. (1978). Rhythmic daily shedding of outer-segment membranes by visual cells in the goldfish. *J. Cell Biol.*, **76**, 593–604.   *90*

OSTERMAN, P. O. and WIDE, L. (1975). The plasma prolactin levels in man during prolongation of darkness in the morning. *Acta Endocrinologica*, **78**, 675–82.   *74*

STRUMWASSER, F. (1965). The demonstration and manipulation of a circadian rhythm in a simple neurone. In *Circadian clocks* (ed. J. Aschoff), pp. 442–62. North Holland Publishing Co., Amsterdam.   *69*

VILLERMET, G. M. and WEALE, R. A. (1969). The optical activity of bleached visual receptors. *J. Physiol.*, **201**, 425–35.   *90*

WEALE, R. A. (1968). Optical activity and the fixation of rods and cones. *Nature (Lond.)*, **220**, 583.   *90*

WEBB, W. B. and AGNEW, H. W. (1975). Sleep efficiency for sleep-wake cycles of varied length. *Psychophysiology*, **12**, 637–41. 65

WEITZMAN, E. D. (1976). Circadian rhythms and episodic hormone secretion in man. *Ann. Rev. Med.*, **27**, 225–43. 75

WEVER, R. (1969). Autonome circadiane Periodik des Menschen unter dem Einfluss verschiedener Beleuchtungsbedingungen. Pflügers Arch., **306**, 71–9. 65–7

YOUNG, R. W. (1967). The renewal of photoreceptor cell outer segments. *J. Cell Biol.*, **33**, 61–72. 82, 85

YOUNG, R. W. (1971a). An hypothesis to account for a basic distinction between rods and cones. *Vision Res.*, **11**, 1–5. 81

YOUNG, R. W. (1971b). The renewal of rod and cone outer segments in the rhesus monkey. *J. Cell Biol.*, **49**, 303–18. 82, 85

YOUNG, R. W. (1977). The daily rhythm of shedding and degradation of cone outer segment membranes in the lizard retina. *J. Ultrastructure Res.*, **61**, 172–85. 89, 90

Chapter 3

ATKINSON, J., BRADDICK, O. and BRADDICK, F. (1974). Acuity and contrast sensitivity of infant vision. *Nature (Lond.)*, **247**, 403–4. 108

ATKINSON, J., BRADDICK, O. and MOAR, K. (1977). Development of contrast sensitivity over the first 3 months of life in the human infant. *Vision Res.* **17**, 1037–44. 109, 110

BACH, L. and SEEFELDER, R. (1914). *Atlas zur Entwicklungsgeschichte des menschlichen Auges*. Verlag von Wilhelm Engelmann, Leipzig and Berlin. 99–104

BARBER, A. N. (1955). *Embryology of the human eve*. Henry Kimpton, London. 94

BLAKEMORE, C., GAREY, L. J. and VITAL-DURANL (1978). Reversal of physiological effects of monocular deprivation in monkeys. *J. Physiol.*, **276**, 47–9P. 128

BOURLIÉRE, F. (1970). The assessment of biological age in man. *Public Health Papers No. 37*, WHO, Geneva. 93

CHERNENKO, G. A. and WEST, R. W. (1976). A re-examination of anatomical plasticity in the rat retina. *J. Comp. Neurol.*, **167**, 49–62. 119

COMFORT, A. (1964). *Ageing: the biology of senescence*. Routledge and Kegan Paul, London. 93

CRAGG, B. G. (1975). The development of synapses in the visual system of the cat. *J. Comp. Neurol.*, **160**, 147–66. 123

DANIELS, J. D., NORMAN, J. L. and PETTIGREW, J. D. (1977). Biases for oriented moving bars in lateral geniculate nucleus neurons of normal and stripe-reared cats. *Exp. Brain Res.*, **29**, 155–72. 119

DAW, N. W., BERMAN, N. E. J. and ARIEL, M. (1978). Interaction of critical periods in the visual cortex of kittens. *Science*, **199**, 565–7. 106, 126

DERRINGTON, A. M. (1978). Development of selectivity in kitten striate cortex. *J. Physiol.*, **276**, 46–7P. 118

DOBSON, V. and TELLER, D. Y. (1978). Visual acuity in human infants: a review and comparison of behavioural and electrophysiological studies. *Vision Res.*, **18**, 1469–83. 110

FISCHER, F. P. (1948). Senescence of the eye. In *Modern trends in ophthalmology* (vol. 2) (ed. A. Sorsby) Butterworth, London. 107

FREEMAN, R. D., MITCHELL, D. E. and MILLODOT, M. (1972). A neural effect of partial visual deprivation in humans. *Science*, **175**, 1384–6. 115, 117

FREEMAN, R. D. and THIBOS, L. N. (1975). Contrast sensitivity in humans with abnormal visual experience. *J. Physiol.*, **247**, 687–710. 115, 116

GUILLERY, R. W. and STELZNER, D. J. (1970). The differential effects of unilateral lid closure upon the monocular and binocular segments of the dorsal lateral geniculate nucleus in the cat. *J. Comp. Neurol.*, **139**, 413–22. 120

GWIAZDA, J., BRILL, S., MOHINDRA, I. and HELD, R. (1978). Infant visual acuity and its meridional variation. *Vision Res.*, **18**, 1557–64.   *109*

HAMILTON, W. J., BOYD, J. D. and MOSSMAN, H. W. (1945). *Textbook of human embryology* (1st edn.). W. Heffer & Sons, Cambridge.   *95*

HEISLER, J. C. (1907). *A text-book of embryology* (3rd edn.). W. B. Saunders, Philadelphia and London.   *97*

HENDRICKSON, A., BOLES, J. and McLEAN, E. B. (1977). Visual activity and behaviour of monocularly deprived monkeys after retinal lesions. *Invest. Ophthal. and Vis. Sci.*, **16**, 469–73.   *129*

HENDRICKSON, A. and KUPFER, C. (1976). The histogenesis of the fovea in the *macaque* monkey. *Invest. Ophthal.*, **15**, 746–56.   *112*

HENKIND, P., BELLHORN, R. W., MURPHY, M. E. and ROA, N. (1975). Development of macular vessels in monkey and cat. *Brit. J. Ophthal.*, **59**, 703–9.   *113*

HIRSCH, H. V. B. and LEVENTHAL, A. G. (1978). Functional modification of the developing visual system. In (vol 9: *Development of sensory systems*) *Handbook of sensory physiology* (ed. M. Jacobson). Springer-Verlag, Berlin.   *105, 118, 119*

HOFFMAN, K. P. and SHERMAN, S. M. (1975). Effects of early binocular deprivation on visual input to cat superior colliculus. *J. Neurophysiol.*, **38**, 1049–59.   *122*

HOWLAND, H. C., ATKINSON, J., BRADDICK, O. and FRENCH, J. (1978). Infant astigmatism measured by photorefraction. *Science*, **202**, 331–3.   *107*

JOHNSON, G. J., MATTHEWS, A. and PERKINS, E. S. (1979). Survey of ophthalmic conditions in a Labrador community. I. Refractive errors. *Brit. J. Ophthal.*, **63**, 440–8.   *130*

KRATZ, K. E., SHERMAN, S. M. and KALIL, R. (1979). Lateral geniculate nucleus in dark-reared cats: loss of Y cells without changes in cell size. *Science*, **203**, 1353–4.   *121*

MAFFEI, L. and FIORENTINI, A. (1976). Monocular deprivation in kittens impairs the spatial resolution of geniculate neurones. *Nature (Lond.)*, **264**, 754–5.   *126*

MANN, I. C. (1928). *The development of the human eye.* Cambridge University Press.   *96–8, 102*

MARSHALL, J. (1978). Ageing changes in human cones. *Proc. 23rd International Congress of Ophthalmology, Kyoto, May 1978*, pp. 375–8. Excerpta Medica, Amsterdam.   *131, 135*

MITCHELL, D. E. (1979). Astigmatism and neural development. *Invest. Ophthal. Vis. Sci.*, **18**, 8–10.   *126*

MOHINDRA, I., HELD, R., GWIAZDA, J. and BRILL, S. (1978). Astigmatism in infants. *Science*, **202**, 329–31.   *107*

SALAPATEK, P. and BANKS, M. S. (1978). Infant sensory assessment: vision. In *Communicative and cognitive abilities; early behavioral assessment* (ed. F. D. Minifie and L. L. Lloyd). University Park Press, Baltimore.   *111*

SPEKREIJSE, H., ESTEVEZ, O. and REITS, D. (1977). Visual evoked potentials and the physiological analysis of visual processes in man. In *Visual evoked potentials in man: new developments* (ed. J. E. Desmedt). Clarendon Press, Oxford.   *111*

VALVERDE, F. (1971). Rate and extent of recovery from dark rearing in the visual cortex of the mouse. *Brain Res.*, **33**, 1–11.   *123*

VAN SLUYTERS, R. C. (1978). Reversal of the physiological effects of brief periods of monocular deprivation in the kitten. *J. Physiol.*, **289**, 1–17.   *126, 127*

VERRIEST, G. (1971). L'influence de l'âge sur les fonctions visuelles de l'homme. *Bull. Acad. R. Med. Belg.*, **11**, 527–77.   *133*

WEALE, R. A. (1963). *The Aging Eye.* H. K. Lewis, London.   *131*

WEALE, R. A. (1964). Comparison of reactions of human and rabbit fundi to photic exposure. *J. Opt. Soc. Amer.*, **54**, 120–6.   *119*

WIESEL, T. N. and HUBEL, D. H. (1974). Ordered arrangement of orientation columns in monkeys lacking visual experience. *J. Comp. Neurol.*, **158**, 307–18.   *124*

WIESEL, T. N. and RAVIOLA, E. (1977). Myopia and eye enlargement after neonatal lid fusion in monkeys. *Nature (Lond.)*, **266**, 66–8.   *129*

WOLFF, E. (1948). *The anatomy of the eye and orbit.* H. K. Lewis, London.   *96*

Chapter 4

BEVERLEY, K. I. and REGAN, D. (1979). Separable after effects of changing-size and motion-in-depth: different neural mechanisms. *Vision Res.*, **19**, 727–32. *167*

BLAKEMORE, C. (1970). A new kind of stereoscopic vision. *Vision Res.*, **10**, 1181–99. *157*

BOWMAKER, J. K. and DARTNALL, H. J. A. (1980). Visual pigments of rods and cones in a human retina. *J. Physiol.*, **298**, 501–11. *140*

BURR, D. C. and ROSS, J. (1979). How does binocular delay give information about depth? *Vision Res.*, **19**, 523–32. *162*

CARPENTER, R. H. S. (1977). *Movements of the eyes.* Pion, London. *146*

CARPENTER, R. H. S. and BLAKEMORE, C. (1973). Interactions between orientations in human vision. *Exp. Brain Res.*, **18**, 287–303. *171*

CHEVREUL, M. -E. (1839). *De la loi du contraste simultané des couleurs et de l'assortiment des objets colorés.* Pitois-Levrault, Paris. *150*

CREUTZFELDT, O. D. and NORTHDURFT, H. C. (1978). Representation of complex visual stimuli in the brain. *Naturwissenschaften*, **65**, 307–18. *170*

DAW, N. W. (1968). Colour-coded ganglion cells in the goldfish retina: extension of their receptive fields by means of new stimuli. *J. Physiol.*, **197**, 567–92. *151*

FLETCHER, B. (1961). *A history of architecture on comparative method* (17th edn.). Athlone Press of the University of London. *176*

GEHRCKE, E. (1948). Neue Versuche über Farbensehen. *Ann. d. Phys.*, **6**, 345–54. *152*

HANSEL, C. E. M. and MAHMUD, S. H. (1978). Comparable retention times for the negative colour after image and the McCollough effect. *Vision Res.*, **18**, 1601–5. *147*

HOMER, W. I. (1964). *Seurat and the science of painting.* MIT Press, Cambridge, Mass. *150*

JULESZ, B. (1971). *Foundations of cyclopean perception.* The University of Chicago Press, Chicago and London. *157, 171*

KALMUS, H. (1965). *Diagnosis and genetics of defective colour vision.* Pergamon Press, Oxford. *143*

LEVINSON, E. and BLAKE, R. (1979). Stereopsis by harmonic analysis. *Vision Res.*, **19**, 73–9. *157, 158*

MAY, J. G., MATTESON, H. H., AGAMY, G. and CASTELLANOS, P. (1978). The effects of differential adaptation on spatial frequency—contingent color after-effects. *Perception and Psychophysics* **23**, 409–12. *147*

McCOLLOUGH, C. (1965). Color adaptation of edge-detectors in the human visual system. *Science*, **149**, 1115–6. *146*

MOLLON, J. D. (1977). The oddity of blue. *Nature (Lond.)*, **268**, 587–8. *145*

MOLLON, J. D. and POLEN, P. G. (1977). An anomaly in the response of the eye to light of short wavelengths. *Phil. Trans. Roy. Soc. Lond. B.*, **278**, 207–40. *145*

MONTAIGNE, M. de (1842). *Apologies for Raymond Sebond* (Chap. 12) (trans. W. Hazlitt). John Templeman, London. *173*

MURCH, G. M. and PAULSON, J. A. (1978). Colorimetric matches of McCollough after-effects. *Vision Res.*, **18**, 365–8. *169*

MÜTZE, K. (1958). *Optik aller Wellenlängen.* Akademie-Verlag, Berlin. *169*

READING, V. M. (1973). An objective correlate of the Pulfrich stereo-illusion. *Proc. R. Soc. Med.*, **66**, 1043–4. *162*

REGAN, D., BEVERLEY, K. and CYNADER, M. (1979). The visual perception of motion in depth. *Scientific American*, **241**, 136–51. *163–6*

RENTSCHLER, I. (1973). Spatial summation in color-receptive pathways. *Vision Res.*, **13**, 325–36. *148*

ROBINSON, J. O. (1972). *The psychology of visual illusion.* Hutchinson University Library, London. *137, 168, 173*

SPERLING, H. G. and HARWETH, R. S. (1971). Red-green cone interactions in the increment-threshold spectral sensitivity of primates. *Science*, **172**, 180–4. *139*

STROMEYER III, C. F. (1972). Edge-contingent color after-effects: spatial frequency specificity. *Vision Res.*, **12**, 717–33. *147*

TYLER, C. W. (1977). Spatial limitations of human stereoscopic vision. *Proc. S.P.I.E.*, **120,** 36–42.   *159*

TYLER, C. W. and SUTTER, E. E. (1979). Depth from spatial frequency difference: an old kind of stereopsis? *Vision Res.*, **19,** 859–65.   *156*

WADE, N. J. (1973). Binocular rivalry and binocular fusion of after-images. *Vision Res.*, **13,** 999–1000.   *155*

WEALE, R. A. (1960). *The eye and its function*. Hatton Press, London.   *142*

WEALE, R. A. (1975). *From sight to light*. Oliver and Boyd, Edinburgh and London. *161*

WEALE, R. A. (1975). Apparent size and contrast. *Vision Res.*, **15,** 945–55.   *178*

WRIGHT, W. D. (1946). *Researches on normal and defective colour vision*. Henry Kimpton, London.   *141*

YOUNG, T. (1802). On the theory of light and colours. *Philosoph. Trans. Roy. Soc. Lond.*, **92,** 20–71.   *140*

ZEKI, S. M. (1974). Cells responding to changing image size and disparity is the cortex of the rhesus monkey. *J. Physiol.*, **242,** 827–41.   *159, 160*

ZEKI, S. M. (1979). Functional specialization and binocular interaction in the visual areas of rhesus monkey prestriate cortex. *Proc. R. Soc. Lond. B.*, **204,** 379–97.   *159*

Index